I0483132

Cancer... A Blessing?

By

Jerry Wilson

Acknowledgements

To all those that have shared this journey...*Especially my friend Neal Griffin.*

To my son Keith, who is my idol, and a special thanks to my beautiful daughter (Kim) for letting me know that expressing my deep, heartfelt, true feelings, with emotion would make this book more effective! I have tried my best to do that. Thank you sweetie!

Is there truly a God? If you ever see a Hummingbird, you know there is a God!

Jerry Wilson's book is testament to the strength, integrity, trust, love, family, friends, good medicine and good medical care that he brought to his diagnosis and treatment, and now fortunately, to his cure and survival. Though treatment has advanced since then, Jerry's book has much to offer any person or family on their own journey through cancer. I highly recommend it!

Elizabeth E. Campbell, M.D.

Dedication…

In loving memory of my beautiful and precious wife, best friend, mentor, and mother of my wonderful children. Irene "Scottie" Williams Wilson, for her unconditional love and support. She was, and will always remain, the glue for our family!

Forward

I have known Jerry Wilson, and his brother Gary, for nearly sixty years. Mentioning both in the same sentence is only natural to me because I have always thought of them kind of as one – The Wilson Twins.

To me, and many other boys who played Little League baseball in Fayetteville, N.C., in the mid-1950's. Jerry and Gary were legends. Both were sensational players, hitting home runs and striking out batters in bunches. I could never tell them apart, neither in looks or ability. One would pitch and the other would catch, meaning the opposition almost always had to face an intimidating Wilson.

Many years later, I got to know the twins as much more than the superb athletes they had been. I found them to be superb men, proud of their Christian faith and glad to talk about Jesus. In fact, both of our daughters think of that aspect when they hear the names Jerry and Gary Wilson.

One Sunday, our family was eating in a restaurant after church, and the Wilsons came to our table to say hello. As they left, they told our girls to always speak up for Jesus, to never be ashamed of Him. They said, "You can't go wrong with Jesus Christ".

In recent years, I have come to know Jerry even

better…like many other folks in Fayetteville, I was aware of his battle with cancer. It was his second time fighting the awful disease.

Over the years, Jerry has encountered numerous health problems. Serious problems. Yet, he was smiling every time I saw him. He wrote blogs in the local newspaper about his experiences, and they were always spiced with humor.

It wasn't that he was not concerned, that he didn't take cancer seriously. He fought hard, and most importantly, he fought with faith. But he knew laughter is a powerful medicine. So he made sure to have plenty of it.

Jerry shared that laughter just as he shared his love and faith for Jesus.

That is what he does in this book.

People write books for a lot of reasons. Fame, money, or a burning desire just to write and tell stories.

Jerry has written this one because he wants to help other people, those diagnosed with cancer and their family members. To tell the truth, though, what he chronicles in the following pages can help anyone.

That's because Jerry is so positive, and his attack on a dreaded disease includes the whole package: faith, courage, commitment, positive thinking and humor…always humor.

He has said that if his book helps one person, then it will be a best-seller in his mind. He will have achieved his goal.

Well, this book will help many people. In my opinion, it will lift every one of us who reads it.

I feel privileged to call Jerry Wilson and Gary Wilson my friends. They are wonderful disciples of Jesus. That is what I think of when I hear their names…even though I will never forget the way they dominated Little League.

This book is going to be a success because it is going to help people live their lives in a stronger, more positive way.

That makes it well worth reading.

Thad Mumau

Preface – Why Write This Book?

So many people have asked me, "Why are you writing a book?" I wanted to answer the question fully for my entire reader audience.

Now a senior in my life's journey (who has frequent "senior moments"), I forget that some folks still use labels. I've been stereotyped as an athlete, a comedian, a twin, a good guy, and not necessarily in that order.

Maybe some people doubt I have the creativity, introspection, or language skills to write a book. (Like my friend, Bill Kirby, Jr…who'll be glad I found out how to turn on my spell checker.) And others might be thinking I plan to celebrate the good and handsome life of Jerry Wilson…I think not!

No, far from it. You will find glimpses of bad and ugly health problems and related life and medical issues in **Cancer…A Blessing?** I have limited the scope here to fighting one major disease twice, Stage 4 Lymphoma (Hodgkin's disease) and cancer of the prostate gland.

I have had a whole gamut of bad and ugly medical problems: several broken bones, total knee replacement, back surgery, bursitis in my left hip, a stint placed in my heart, glaucoma and total blindness in my right eye, plus the two bouts with cancer. But I will not bore you with all that.

For readers who just want a short answer about why I wrote this book, I hope my experiences show that how each and every person responds to a crisis can affect the outcome of any health crisis.

The first reason for writing is to help others. I hope my words and experiences can create a tool or strategy to help control, prevent, or cope with health issues (and resulting life disruptions).

I am hoping to do more than to share a tool. I want to offer readers a secret weapon: **attitude**. As I fought my battles, **attitude** was my most important weapon. As the saying goes, *an ounce of prevention is worth a pound of cure.* I'm saying that **attitude** is like an ounce of prevention, or precaution, which is worth pounds (or years) of good health.

My second reason for writing is to honor my wife, Mrs. Irene "Scottie" Williams Wilson, for whom a sudden illness was fatal.

Scottie Wilson appeared to be one of the healthiest women I had ever known. None of us suspected there was scar tissue wrapped around her intestines, silently causing sepsis and slowly killing intestines and other organs. Scottie was literally poisoned to death by her own body. Sick one day…suddenly, gone the next.

Scottie stood by me through many medical problems. Her love and support extended my life. I think this book also is partly from Scottie's heart to you

My third reason for writing is to praise and acknowledge the Lord of my life, Jesus Christ. After being treated by many doctors, I know that Jesus Christ is the Great Physician. Having Him as my friend, surrendering to His will, and believing His Word were important in keeping my **attitude** about my health.

Besides my belief in Jesus' healing power and love, I know the support and prayers of many loving people were also tools in my battles.

Medical Disclaimer

I am not a medical doctor, nor have I had any medical training, nor do I hold any type of medical degree. The views and opinions stated in **Cancer...A Blessing?** are simply my opinions, and should NEVER be interpreted as specific medical advice, and must be used only as general information. Consult a qualified medical professional (As I did) regarding any medical issues.

I have been treated at, driven by, or just visited in the following medical centers:

Proton Treatment Center, University of Florida, Jacksonville, FL

Duke Medical Center, Durham, NC

University of North Carolina Medical Center, Chapel Hill, NC

Rex Cancer Center, Raleigh, NC

Bowman Gray School of Medicine, Winston-Salem, NC

Cancer Center of Cape Fear Valley Medical Center, Fayetteville, NC

Cancer Centers of North Carolina, Raleigh, NC and Dunn, NC

Contents

Etc…

Chapter 1

In The Beginning

(Kind of Biblical... you think?)

Hopefully many will read this book. Hopefully they will find something that will be helpful while fighting some type of cancer...that is truly my goal. But for those of you that don't know me, I want to share just a little of myself. I honestly feel it will give some insight as to the inner side of me and my thought processes, as well as, help someone endure the pain.

My brother Gary and I were born in Beaufort, North Carolina; and I was the first born of identical twins. (Therefore entitling me to the family fortune, being the first born son). Our childhood home is now listed as a historic site...with a special historical marker on the front of the house. My granddad worked at the old mill in Beaufort, where he repaired equipment. I really don't know if my grandparents were buying the home or renting it. If I had to guess as to what the home cost in those days, my guess would be around the three thousand range. Today it is valued at over $600,000. Sadly, this fine home is not part of the Wilson estate.

Granddad passed away from a brain tumor when Gary and I were about four years old. As I recall, sometime the following year we moved to Fayetteville to live with our grandmother, Rossie Barnhill. We always called her mother, even though she was our grandmother. Mother raised us with love and Christian values that shaped our identity. We had intangible blessings that money couldn't buy. I normally refer to her as the person that introduced me to this wonderful Carpenter. She actually introduced Him to many people. She taught Sunday school for more years that I can remember.

On a side note, a few years back, I decided to get into politics. I ran for City Council here in Fayetteville, NC...what a learning experience that was. One night all the candidates attended a dinner at Highland Country Club which was sponsored by the State Certified Public Accounts Association. Each candidate had about eight minutes to talk. The first thing I said as I stood before them was this..."I'm going to be honest and tell you up front of a problem I had as a young person growing up. You will find out about it sooner or later and I want you to hear it from me...I had a drug problem, a very serious drug problem as a youth."

Well, you could have heard a pin drop. Had there been flies in the room, they would have had a field day filling all the wide open mouths. "Yes, I had a drug problem, we were DRUG to church every time the door was open!" I will always be eternally grateful for how mother gave her life for my brother and me, and for introducing me to a Man we know as the Carpenter.

By the way, my first and last involvement in politics was unsuccessful...and it was probably for the best! My dear friend (Bill Thames) once told me, "Three people told you to run and Three thousand could have not talked you out of it"........maybe true!

Growing up, our home at 2116 Rock Avenue in Fayetteville, NC, was on a dirt road. I still remember our Rock Avenue phone number over sixty years later…484-0408. In those good old days everyone on our street had a telephone party line, and you got "on line" when you could. By the time we were teenagers, Fayetteville Senior High School (now called Terry Sanford High School) had been built almost in our back yard. Imagine the hardship: We had to walk almost 300 yards to school…really bad on cold, rainy days. And forget it, if it ever snowed! Speaking of snowing, Gary and I had a paper routes for over six years and I hated delivering on days of ice and snow. During that six year period, we amassed over $600.00 in the bank. What a stash!

I went to school at Westlawn Elementary, and then Alexander Graham Jr. High, which was down town. In 1963 graduating from Fayetteville Senior High School with some 320 others.

I was an average student, but I did not like homework. Studying was not my best subject, which I have regretted to this day. Well, Gary and I did study piano three years, along with two of our buddies at the time, Frank Maynard and George Breece. To this day, I can still play "America" and "Joshua Fit the Battle of Jericho." I have brief downer moments about those piano lessons taken from Ms. Cook. See, I have never, ever been asked to play either of those tunes at one single party or church function.

Since age nine, or maybe earlier, I was involved in sports. Anything to do with a ball had top priority. My world in Jr. High, and high school was just sports (well maybe girls also). Competition – winning and not losing – were very important to me.

Most of my time, interest and energy went into practicing and playing football, basketball and baseball. I think my extra efforts paid off. There are only three undefeated football teams in the history of the school, ours was one of them. Not only were we tough, but also, we played without a star. Our fierce teamwork not only served our school; but also, it prepared me for life…along with the other sports. Without a star, we were a more cohesive team and played as a team…Go Bulldogs!

I was awarded a full baseball scholarship to Southwood Junior College where I completed my associate's degree in 1965. (Pistol Pete Maravich also attended this school a few years later) At the same time the baseball coach at East Carolina University was finalizing plans to recruit me, when I was badly hurt in a double header in Greenville against East Carolina University. I was run over on a squeeze play by the runner on third. He was a HUGE guy who was the starting fullback on the ECU football team, I never played another game of baseball after that injury (broken collar bone)…but I still have the wounds to show for it! Believe me!

That's not entirely true. Years later, shortly after joining a church in Atlanta, I saw in the bulletin one Sunday that they were having practice and tryouts for the Men's softball team. Being the star athlete I was, I felt this would be an opportunity for exercise and a chance to get to meet some of the men in the church.
Because of my total blindness (due to glaucoma) in my right eye, I could not tell if the ball was six yards from me, or three feet from me. I had Spalding marks all over my stomach and chest! (From the ball hitting me.) At that very moment I asked God if he would get me off that field safely and able to walk, I would never go back on a baseball or softball field again. I still have the pair of Louisville Slugger softball shoes that have only been worn once! Size 11 if anyone is interested.

Beating cancer went into the win column, and I hope the zero remains in the lost column. Anyway, I guess I will never be in the hall of fame for beating cancer. Bobby Richardson, the great second baseman for the New York Yankees, put it so well. He said he always wanted to be in the baseball hall of fame, but it was far more important to be in God's Hall of Fame, how true…and I know I will make that one! Also, had I not had that injury, the likes of Yogi Berra, Elston Howard, Roy Campanella and Johnny Bench would not have had a prayer in the big leagues, had I been able to go on to the majors….I think not! They all were my idols back then, when young men had real idols. The sports idols of today often use some type of strength-building drugs. What does that teach anyone, and who really wants a role model on drugs. And just think, what would life be like without the guidance and clever life supporting sayings from Yogi such as: *"When you get to fork in the road…take it"*, or *"No one goes to that restaurant anymore because you can't get a seat"*, what great advice for life! Sure has helped me over the years, especially just going out to dinner.

Anyway, back to that baseball accident that happened at East Carolina. I took the lemons and made lemonade! Almost immediately I met the love of my life, the beautiful Irene Scottie Williams.

I met her in October of 1966, while visiting my brother during Greek week at Atlantic Christian College. Scottie was enrolled there and was studying to receive an English degree. Our first date was for lunch on Sunday.

She said, if I would go to church with her and her sorority, she would go to lunch with me…let's see, sitting with thirty plus girls and then lunch with Scottie, a no brainer, you think?

I proposed to Scottie the week after I met her. I gave her a ring at Christmas. We were then married on June 11, 1967. My dear friend, Ronnie Collins always said that I seemed to always know what I wanted.

I was working with the Fayetteville Observer selling display advertising. With that job, I had the opportunity to make $10,000 a year, and I did. (Big money huh? Believe it or not, it was back then.) I was driving a slick navy blue 1966 Mustang as a bachelor. I was a member of Green Valley Country Club here in Fayetteville, I thought I was on top of the world!

After getting married, Scottie and I settled here in Fayetteville into a house on Glenville Avenue. The house came with a whopping $9,800 price tag. With a big whopping monthly payment of almost $79. I had to resign my membership in the Country Club. After that I traded my beautiful Mustang in for a more practical Volkswagen Beetle. We then settled into being one happy family...the two of us.

Most of my career was in the office equipment business:

Xerox Corporation, Eastman Kodak Company and IKON. Scottie and I could never have guessed that we would move so many times.

We enjoyed turning several different houses into homes filled with love and many blessings. We lived in Asheville NC; Greensboro NC, where my children were born; Raleigh NC; Rochester NY; Atlanta Ga.; and Raleigh NC. We finally came full circle, returning to Fayetteville.

Technology was rapidly changing everything when I decided to retire at the age of 59. About that time, Scottie was asked what it was like, being married to me for all those years (44). Her response was, "It has been a good ride." Maybe she said that because we had lived in so many places and have literally traveled all over the United States together. I would take her on numerous business trips with me. She loved Boston and NY.

People thought Scottie was an excellent conversationalist. No, not a talker. She asked questions and let *you* do all the talking. She just listened and learned.

She was an avid reader, often going through up to three or more books a week. I only hope she would have enjoyed reading this book!

National politics was a game to her; and she was as politically astute as anyone I have ever met, man or woman! She could talk the talk, and walk the walk politically with the best of them.

One of Scottie's favorite scripture verses was Matthew 25:40...*Inasmuch as ye have done it unto one of the least of these, my brethren, ye have done it unto me.*" She put family and others before self. She was the glue that kept our family together and running. She was generous, strong, beautiful, and intelligent. Scottie taught me more than any professor ever taught me...oh, so much more.

Maybe the most important thing was she let me know the sun did not rise and set on my backside! By that I mean, others were more important, regardless of how big or small. From her I learned that the only way to have a friend is to be a friend. On top of all her wonderful qualities, she was a tremendous judge of character. She liked a person for his/her character and values, not who they were. So many of us need work in this area.

As you can imagine, I miss Scottie – my precious wife, friend, and mentor of 44 years. I am still working through her unexpected passing in 2011. As I type this now, big tears are rolling down my cheeks.

Just days after Scottie's passing, I got a call from the president of her company expressing condolences. A few days later, one of the greeters at her workplace she called on telephoned to say how much Scottie meant to her. To anyone, that says volumes and volumes!

Some say life is not fair. It does seem unfair that Scottie did not get to teach and guide the very ones she loved most, her grandchildren.

While there's a special place in my heart reserved for Scottie, I am thankful to have our two wonderful children, Keith and Kimberly, and our three adorable grandchildren, Elizabeth Grace, Luke and Caden....Scottie cut the umbilical cord at Caden's birth. They all have their nana Scottie's good looks and brains.

Readers, remember to love and enjoy the ones you are with...because you never know when God might call them home.

At this writing in 2013, the Bulldogs of Fayetteville High (Terry Sanford now) have marked yet another milestone, celebrating the 100th anniversary of the school's founding. And to celebrate the 50th Reunion of the Class of '63, some classmates again walked those halls in July 2013 –this time as mellow seniors. That's another full circle, don't you think: The one hundred who attended were surprised by how many from our classmates are deceased...a reminder how important our health is.

The reunion also got me to thinking seriously about trying to encourage other people by sharing my experiences. And that's how the idea began for **Cancer...A Blessing?**

Chapter 2

Cancer, The Beginning

At 52, I had a beautiful family and had had a very good career. We were living the good life (the stuff about which this book is not written!) Except for some broken bones, I had stayed fit and enjoyed good health. I was comfortable in my identity (I had been away from Fayetteville long enough [30 plus years] that people would refer to me as Jerry, not which twin are you)…enjoyed a reputation for being fun-loving, cool, laid back, just a normal, all around good guy, some might say.

Time to move to Raleigh. We had not sold the house in Atlanta, so Scottie stayed there while I started work in Raleigh. Years earlier, Scottie studied and obtained her broker's license which worked out well with all the moves we had made over the years. She knew all the ins and outs of the real estate business which helped us a great deal. Not to mention the money she saved us from not having to pay real estate broker's fees, etc…

Our longtime friends, Bill and Sandra Faison offered me a place to stay in Raleigh when I began my new job. Needless to say, this was a God-send at the time. Bill and I have been friends for a number of years and he is probably the easiest person in the world to talk with. An interesting point here is, with all I was going through…very, very sick, we never talked about it specifically.

We had numerous conversations about life in general (Especially golf) and only discussed cancer if I brought it up. In my opinion, that's a good way to deal with someone suffering any type of illness that you are around for any length of time. Be yourself, and treat the one that is ill as if it's just a normal day. Just your presence alone, will bring great joy to anyone suffering from cancer.

Of course, shortly after moving to Raleigh I got very sick. As I recall, the symptoms began as fevers, major night sweats, fatigue, weakness, and exhaustion. They hung on, and hung on and hung on.

I did not have an established family doctor at the time, so I stopped by what I call a "doctor in a box" for a checkup. I do not recall the doctor's name, but she was Swedish and very tall, maybe 5'11" or more. ("Dr. Tall-Swede" and her husband (a doctor also) were co-owners of their business and were doing quite well.) Dr. Tall-Swede diagnosed a very bad upper respiratory issue. She put me on some antibiotics.

A few weeks later, the antibiotics still were not working. So I went back in to see the "Tall-Swede" in the box. She put me on stronger antibiotics. After a few more weeks, those still had not worked either. Starting to worry now…still feeling lousy and getting uptight.

Make a note now, readers, that people in my support group have challenged me to be honest and tell my real emoticns. See? I'm trying. You also must be aware that I get emotional at grand openings of 7-11 stores.

Anyway, finally Dr. Tall-Swede referred me for a *computerized tomography* scan, or CT scan. At the time, I had never had a CT scan. I could not imagine being trapped in a huge metal circular device, not allowed to move. Just the thought of it kept me strung out for days. Well, the scan turned out to be a piece of cake, no problem at all.

After a week or so, the scan results were back. I was not pleased at all…well, *shocked* is more like what I felt. Dr. Tall-Swede showed me that there were *lesions* in my body in numerous locations. She tried to soften the blow a bit by saying they all were small in size. They looked like they were everywhere to me at the time.

I was referred to Dr. Elizabeth Campbell, an *Oncologist* in Raleigh. (Dr. Elizabeth Campbell, MD graduated from Duke School of Medicine in 1982 and has been practicing for over 30 years now.) My two personal nurses were Lisa Childress and Jennifer Sneac. They were, and still are my two special angels!

Well, I don't have a medical degree (even though I played a doctor on TV once…just kidding). But I knew what seeing an oncologist meant. Dr. Elizabeth Campbell was a pleasant surprise. She was the consummate professional that I was about to turn my life over to!

During the early stages of my treatment she was blessed with twins, her first two children. I told her it must have been some sort of osmosis from me, since I was a twin. We both enjoyed the laugh.

The beginning, yes, and I was not just fearful. I was falling apart and scared for my life. And that's where it all began!

Chapter 3

Diagnosis and Shock

There are three words we all like to hear: "I *love you*". But there are also three words we never want to hear in our life time: "*You have cancer*".

I used to think of cancer as something that you heard about or read about in the newspaper…not something that could ever happen to me. You know, Aunt Susie has cancer or Mr. Jones, down the street has cancer, but not me.

I had a lump in my neck. When Dr. Campbell saw me for the first time, the very first thing she said was, "*that needs to come out.*"

So now surgery was involved! And the surgeon was not encouraging at all. No, he painted a very bad picture. I can remember his words to this day as he was looking down my throat with his hose, I mean scope. He said, "*That looks ugly, not good at all, I wish I had better news for you.*" Stress city…losing my cool Scottie was with me and heard the very same words but later said, it's ok, Dr. Campbell will take care of everything…Scottie was always encouraging, always comforting. She was my life support system!

After surgery, the specimen was sent to pathology. Because of my age, the doctors had the biopsy read and reviewed several times. As I understand it, Hodgkin's is easier to treat and is also known as a young person's disease. (I always thought I was younger than what my birth certificate says...there must be an error on my birth certificate). They, the pathologist, thought it had to be a mistake because Hodgkin's is more commonly found in younger people.

Hearing the medical diagnosis for cancer that morning, I think I briefly slipped into shock...still unsure how I got back to the Faison's home. My body seemed numb, almost in a blur or a trance. Was this just a bad dream? Unfortunately, not!

When Sandra Faison came home for lunch that day, she saw me sitting limp and pale...almost what they call a catatonic state, close to a zombie sitting on the couch in the living room. Sandra was the very first person to hear about my diagnosis. She was worried about my state of mind and she didn't go back to work that day. From the start, she was a key person of my support group.

No, it was not a bad dream. It was real. As I began snapping back to near-normal, thoughts came racing into my head. I begin to think: *How much longer do I have? How do I tell the ones I love so dearly? How do I tell my wife? How do I tell my children? How will they all get along after I am gone? Are all my financial matters in order? Hey, I don't even have a will? (My friend Bill Senter took care of that).*

Telling my family was the worst, or one of the worst experiences in my entire life. Tears, oh, so many tears! Fear. Heartache and pain...almost unbearable, like my heart was just breaking in half. Now even more thoughts began to pop up in my head: *Was I ready for death? What would death be like? And, did I deserve to go to heaven?*

A pastor and friend at the time was Dr. David Crocker, pastor at Snyder Memorial Baptist Church. His response was timely and just what I wanted and needed to hear. David said, *"None of us deserves to go to heaven. We all will get there through the loving grace of God, simply by believing"*.

More questions: *Would I turn into a vegetable and have to be nursed daily? Would I be vomiting every day from the chemo? (I never vomited once during the entire chemo process!).* So many thoughts. Only someone who has been told he/she has cancer can really understand the jumbled feeling. I hope and pray none of you reading this material will have to go through this major health issue.

On a lighter note. Since I started taking chemo in September of 1996, Christmas was just around the corner. I have always taken pride in looking my very best in a nice suit and tie for work...shoes shined of course. Well, for Christmas, Scottie, Keith and Kimberly thought it would be nice to get me a navy blue Brooks Brothers suit. I had, at the time, never owned a Brooks Brother suit. As I was opening my present, the three of them were very anxious to see my reaction. When I finally got it opened, I started balling like a baby. Tears were everywhere. (No Kleenex here, bring me the towel) They wanted to know what was wrong, they all thought I would enjoy this suit.

Well, I did enjoy the suit, in fact very much. However, my first reaction after seeing it was they had bought me something nice to be buried in. They all knew I was going to die, but no one was telling me the truth. Why were they keeping the truth from me? Years later I have really had a good laugh over that one, but must admit, it took some time!

Chapter 4

Fighting Lymphoma (Hodgkin's)

There are two types of lymphoma: Hodgkin's disease and non-Hodgkin's Disease. The good news (if you can call it that) was mine was Hodgkin's disease, which is a cancer of the white blood cells. I have been told Hodgkin's is also a disease that normally affects younger people and is easier to treat. I have no medical knowledge of that, however.

The bad news was, it had spread. Lesions were everywhere (in the upper and lower diaphragm). I was in stage 4. Stage 5 is your local funeral home! (No, NOT going yet...too much to do!) At the time I was told or read somewhere that Stage 4 Hodgkin's patient's had about a 27 percent chance of survival!

I was diagnosed in September 1996 and treatments started the same month. A port was put into the right side of my chest for receiving the chemotherapy. The needle used to stick into the port was called a *bumble-bee* because it stung like the devil. OH, yes, it did.

Chemotherapy, or chemo, is referred to as a *cocktail by some*, because it is a mixture of several drugs. I think the mixture was Adriamycin, which was red in color. I do not remember the other drugs but I am sure there was an anti-nausea mixture in the cocktail.

While I was waiting to get my port put in and take my first chemo session, I had some very good news come from work. Because of the amount of sales my sales team had produced, we had won a trip to St. Croix. I accepted the good news with mixed emotions. Here I was sick as a dog, but wanted to take Scottie on this trip…she deserved it! St Croix is one of the most beautiful places I have ever visited…it was unbelievably beautiful. Maybe the clearest water in the world and scenery that post cards are made of. Our suite was incredible, it had one large bedroom, den and sitting area, plus a small kitchen area. The most amazing shower I have ever seen, it must have been ten by ten in size. You could have put an army in there.

On my next visit to see Dr. Campbell, I asked if I could reschedule my first chemo session so I could take Scottie to St. Croix. Her response was, "sure, go ahead and have a wonderful time". Well, we went. Unfortunately my illness made it a not so wonderful trip. Oh it was beautiful beyond words, but I had something like heavy flu conditions that were not ideal for travel, especially the night sweats. In fact I don't have the proper words to describe how miserable they were. I would wake up two or three times during the night and would have to change clothes and sheets they were so wet. (We made the hotel aware of my condition and plenty of sheets were on hand).

One morning while we were there I woke up and looked out the window and saw a beautiful area by the water where I could go sit and watch the day come in. I also wanted a place I could just be alone to pray (and oh yes, cry and have my own little pity party).

Naturally I took a towel with me, not to dry off, but rather to use as my Kleenex. For some reason, I was planning on having quite a few tears.

As I sat there in all that beauty I looked down and saw a stone that got my attention. It was beautiful and very smooth. As I picked it up, a calmness came over me as if something warm had just been put into my blood stream. I accepted that stone as a gift from God, and kept as a reminder of that special moment. I still have that stone in my possession to this day.

Now, why did I tell you this story and how does it relate in any way to this book. The reason is this…I postponed the chemo session to go on the trip…right? As soon as I got back and had my first chemo session, the night sweats went away a day or two later and never returned. Maybe this will help someone else in their decision making process towards taking chemo. Also, keep in mind, everyone reacts differently to different types of chemo. One of the nurses told me that two people, taking exactly the same chemo cocktail, could have two completely different reactions.

A bad example of the above paragraph happened one day while I was in Dr. Campbell's office for a chemo treatment. One of the nurses asked me, *"Since you are our poster cancer boy and have the type of attitude that you have, will you call my brother in Wilmington and talk with him? He has the exact same thing you have, but is only a stage two, I believe you could lift him up a bit and hopefully change his attitude."* I did give him a call and it was not good. The world was against him and his attitude was at a 0 out of a possible 10.

Three months or so down the road I was in for another treatment. I purposely asked the nurse that had asked me to call her brother how he was doing. Her response was, *"Jerry, he passed away last week!"* I turned white as a sheet and could hardly stand from the weakness in my knees. How could this happen, he was only a stage 2 and I was a stage 4. That's when she shared with me how different people react to the same chemo with the same disease and have different results. It, to say the least, opened my eyes to how important overall attitude affects ones outcome.

I would go in on Mondays for treatment that lasted about four hours. Tuesdays usually went fine, somewhat normal for about a day and a half. Boy, the cocktail could kick butt! It sure did mine. Around noon on Wednesday, I would get the side effects – hiccups, flushing in the face, and nausea. I would be home in the bed for two or three days, weak, tired, miserable...eating very little. Nothing had any flavor, and food odors were repulsive. A little taste of hell, it seemed.

It is important that your white cell count remain good. A drop or low count could prohibit you from taking a chemo treatment session.

At one point, my white count became lower...To help keep it up, I had to give myself shots daily to rebuild the white count to standard. Boy, did I throw another pity party when I found out this news.

Lisa was showing me how to give myself a shot and she asked me to pull my pants down. Immediately I said, *"You just want to see me in my boxers"*...after telling me how silly I was, she said she had been giving herself shots for years now. She was diabetic. Obviously that made the process of giving myself shots a little less important. The shots were not that bad, but the side effects could be quiet painful. Because of the pain one week, I decided to skip a few shots, when I showed up for chemo, my white count was below standard to take my chemo treatment.

Without a doubt, that was the last time I skipped giving myself shots, regardless of any amount of pain. Lisa, being diabetic reminded me of the saying...I used to complain because I had no shoes until I saw a man who had no feet. I was taught a very valuable lesson that day. For you golfers, it also makes those three footers so totally un-important!

The worse I felt, the more I believed the chemo was working harder to kill cancer cells (just a personal thought). Usually I would start to feel better just in time for the next treatment! And that was the routine repeated every other week for, I believe, around seven or eight months, I honestly can't remember.

I remember saying to Dr. Campbell one day, *"there sure are a lot of sick people in the chemo room"*, she whispered back to me, *"yes, but you are not one of them"*. An example of compassion, positive attitude and a boost for me at the right time. Dr. Campbell was my hero then and is to this day.

Oh, and the hair thing. One day I bet Dr. Campbell that I would not lose my hair, she eagerly accepted the bet...a gentleman's bet. I knew I was going to lose as quickly as she accepted the bet!!! Yes, I lost the bet and lost most of all my scalp hair. Hair loss affects all parts of your body, not just the top of your head. If you are vain at all (and I am, but just a little...) well, chemo might help you get past that minor flaw.

During this period, one day I got out of the shower and jumped from fright at what I saw in the mirror.
 I thought a 12-year-kid had come into the bathroom and was staring at me! I just didn't recognize myself naked and without any hair....anywhere!

Continuing on a lighter note:
I remember reading about some research being done on how a sense of humor can affect our health in a good way. (I'm thinking it was written by a comedian, but wouldn't that be a conflict of interest?)

Well, as I mentioned earlier, the chemo cocktail was red. My nurse Lisa had told me not to be alarmed if my urine was a somewhat pink or reddish. Chemo would cause a change in the color. During my very first chemo session, my twin brother, Gary was visiting with me. Well, when I had to go to the bathroom, Gary helped me push the chemo cart into the bathroom and helped make sure I did not stumble or fall.

Just as Gary and I came back out, Lisa came into the chemo room. Gary decided to have some fun with her. With a real straight face and serious tone, he said, "Jerry's urine looked normal. But actually, it was mine that was a little reddish. What's that all about?" I took a second or two for that to set in with her. Then we all three burst out laughing. Laughter...the best medicine...you think?

A tool from Ace Hardware…I'm sure. During the chemo process, occasionally the oncologist will explore the bone marrow to see if the cancer cells have spread to that area. It's called a bone marrow biopsy. I have heard of people having a bone marrow transplant to help cure their cancer, but I was not familiar with the process at all. I did know that most patients have to go on a search to find a matching bone marrow donor. I was not concerned about that because I had a perfect match in my twin brother. Had we had to do it, I'm sure my brother would have charged me a reasonable price for his!

Dr. Campbell scheduled a bone marrow biopsy for me and I never gave it a second thought. The bone marrow is extracted from your hip bone and I figured it would be a zip-zip and I would be out of there…not hardly. In order to get to the bone marrow, I swear she used a tool from Ace Hardware, and a big one at that. Thank goodness it didn't have an engine on it, or maybe if it had it would have been easier to inject! During the process of this tool being in my back, people said they could hear me whining and screaming from miles away, maybe all the way to the coast. I don't doubt it at all.

GOOD NEWS…no cancer in my bone marrow.
A few months later it was time for another bone marrow biopsy. Scottie was not with me during the first procedure. She was there this time and I told her she might want to stay outside. It, I'm sure, was not going to be a pretty sight and being the wimp that I am, I really didn't want her to see me cry.

When Lisa (my nurse) came to prep me for this second procedure I asked and begged her for a lot of juice (pain killer). Lisa said she would check with Dr. Campbell and fortunately the Dr. approved it. Also, Scottie being the trooper she was said she would be in the room with me for comfort and encouragement. By the time the Dr. got into the room, I was on cloud nine, and could not shut up from talking (of course I had no idea what I was saying), I believe I talked the whole time the procedure was going on, telling jokes etc.. Dr. Campbell went into one side of my back and then the other side for good measure I guess. Heck, she could have gone in-between my eyes and it would have not mattered one bit. This biopsy also turned out to be negative. There were no other visits to Ace Hardware...thank you Lord.

A few weeks down the road while having a checkup, Dr. Campbell told me her dad was a doctor also. She said she used the same amount of juice (pain killer) that her dad used to use when setting a broken bone...I owe her dad a big thank you very much! I'm sure he is a wonderful doctor.

Cancer and chemo has its side effects, one of them is the heart. Of course, this depends on the type of chemo or cocktail you are taking, and the amount that has to be administered to you. It can even cause some type of heart disease. After taking my treatments for some time, Dr. Campbell sent me in for a test to be done on my heart. I am not sure what the test or procedure is called but it went something like this. You lay on a table with a bicycle wheel and they told me that I would be peddling for three minutes and then he would make it a little more difficult the next three minutes and so on. That seemed easy enough. Just before he got started his nurse came in and absolutely blew me away. I don't know if she was an angel or not, but she sure looked like one. Beautiful as the day is long.

Here I lay on this table with basically no hair, looking like I had yellow jaundice from the chemo and weighing in at about 160 lbs. (skinny)…not a pretty site. However, in spite of all this, I was going to do my best to impress this beautiful young lady.

The first three minutes went ok and I am so sure this young nurse was very impressed with me. Then the doctor tightened up the wheel…a little more difficult. The next six minutes I thought I was going to die, but would not show it for fear it may have shown some weakness on my part to this beautiful nurse.

Well, I went home and told my lovely wife Scottie about the experience and we both had a good laugh…side effect, I could hardly walk for about a day and a half.

Chapter 5

Attitude

After the treatments and scans were completed in 1997, I met with Dr. Campbell about my official prognosis. She said, "Jerry, we cannot find anymore cancer." After that news I could not hold back the tears! I believe I remember that even her eyes became a little teary also.

This surprises me, and maybe it will you also: During my ordeal with lymphoma, I never said once, *why did this happen to me?* But after hearing Dr. Campbell's news, I said, "Lord, why me"???? Why was He so good to me, to allow my healing to manifest?

Writing this now in 2013, I am thinking about some of the teachings by our senior pastor at Snyder Memorial Baptist Church in Fayetteville NC, the Reverend John Cook. The pastor taught about prayer several Sundays ago, including suggested prayer positions. For example, Jesus even prayed lying down

Well, my bout with cancer taught me the value of prayer. It also forced me into a new prayer position – down on my knees. My crisis taught me submission. It also taught me the value of praise and thanksgiving. Getting good news like "no cancer" can bring you to your knees. I don't care how big and tough you might be! Yes, speaking from personal experience that brought me to my knees. I was overwhelmed by God's mercy and love for me.

Those were tears of joy. It had been a long, miserable ordeal and an incredible fight…but we had won (we being God, Dr. Campbell, Me and Scottie).

Thanks to a lot of prayer, God's help, a good doctor, and great medicine, I had beaten cancer! No death sentence. No funeral home.

My great grandmother raised eleven children. (Unfortunately, buried 7 of them) She was the salt of the earth and I loved her dearly. I remember two important things about her, her strong faith and her beautiful smile. As she (and I got older), I enjoyed her reaction every time I gave her a big bear hug, telling her, "I love hugging big breasted women". My teasing her brought that unforgettable smile to her face.

I think my thoughts have affected my personality. I try to stay upbeat with a smile on my face. That smile (Like my great grandmothers) has two purposes: first, it is contagious; and second, it makes people wonder what I'm up to!

My sense of humor has opened doors and has made life more enjoyable. It seems to have a healing affect.

I can carry a conversation. When I volunteer, I try to be genuine with people and to show interest in their thoughts, asking open-ended questions. (Questions that require more than just a yes or no) It helps to show humor, love, and hope. It is especially effective while visiting patients in a chemo room.

A friend told me about recent research by Dr. Caroline Leaf, an Australian neuropsychologist. It shows that our brain communicates with every cell in our body thousands of times each day. Also, negative or "toxic thoughts" can have harmful effects on our brains and our overall health. Yes, I think our bodies respond to positive words and beliefs, or thoughts. Our thoughts and our words affect our health and reflect our attitude.

Look at Proverbs 17:22 – "A cheerful heart is good medicine". Sounds like the secret weapon – attitude! And what about Proverbs 23:7? "As a man thinketh in his heart, so is he." God knew what he was doing.....works for me.

Another story, lighter side of attitude...
On one of my visits back for a checkup, Scottie saw a lady getting hooked up for her first chemo session. Always thinking of others, Scottie talked me into going over to try and cheer her up. The lady really looked like she was on a big downer. Well, she was.

I walked over and said, *"Hey, it's a piece of cake."* The lady gave a curt and angry response to me, *"How would you know"?* At that point, the nurse introduced us and told her I had been through the same ordeal and treatments. We had a general conversation for several minutes. Then I leaned over and said in a whisper, *"Neither the doctors or nurses will tell you this. But when I first started chemo, I was not this pretty. But look how pretty chemo has made me!* (Even with a small amount of hair). She joined me in a really good laugh!

As I was walking away, the lady said to me, *"Mr. Wilson, I don't mind looking pretty like you, but will it make me a nut also?"* Again, we all laughed out loud. I often wonder how she made out, but I'll bet she is doing fine today...I sure hope so!

I love this anonymous quote about attitude: *Your life today is the result of your attitude and the decisions you made yesterday. Your life tomorrow will be the result of your attitude and decisions you make today.*

I have never not enjoyed being around a person with a great attitude. It is somewhat contagious. Attitude is so very important, not only in cancer treatments, but also in our daily lives as well. I know, from my experience, that attitude can increase a person's chances of beating cancer also!

Chapter 6

Message From God

Another story…Maybe my all-time favorite!
We were very close to our Atlanta neighbors, Downey
and Sondra Walker. The Walkers invited Scottie and me
to attend their church, Mount Bethel United Methodist
Church. We liked the pastor, Dr. Randy Mickler, who
was an awesome speaker. After attending several
Sundays, we joined the church.

Every year or so, Randy gave a sermon about how he
had received a personal message from God when his
mother passed away. Mrs. Mickler, his mother, had been
a member of the church for a long time. Randy
remembered how, as a child, he had often asked,
"Mother, how do I know there is a God?" Mrs. Mickler
would answer, "*Son, if you ever see a hummingbird, you will
know there is a God.*" Her reasoning was that these small
birds should not even be able to fly because of their wing
size. Only through the grace of God, could they fly.

Eventually, Randy felt called to enter seminary to become a minister. While he was there his mother passed away. The new minister at the church did not know his mother very but Randy wanted the service conducted by someone who knew Mrs. Mickler. He concluded he would conduct the service, but he wondered if he would have the courage and composure in this time of grief. Right up to the day of the service, Randy still worried unsure about what to do.

No flowers were blooming as Randy stood gazing out the window prior to the service for his mother. From out of nowhere a hummingbird hovered in front of him at the window! To Randy it was a message of assurance about proceeding with his mother's service. (Although he did not tell us, I imagine Randy did a terrific job with the service to celebrate his mother's life….and I'm sure she would have been very proud of him.)

Why did I tell this story? Because it reminds me of how God sent me a very similar personal message. As you recall, my prognosis for Hodgkin's disease, Stage 4 was a very low survival chance of about 27 percent.

When I was going through chemo, I would go in every so often for a CT (computerized thermography) scan to see how the chemo was working. Well, near the end of my chemo treatments, I had a week off after my scan. I tried to work a few days during the break. Lisa, the nurse called me and said she had the preliminary results of my scan.

For whatever the reason, I did not have a warm, fuzzy feeling about getting those results. I can't explain why, I just didn't. I asked Lisa to give me a few minutes to run home, then to call me there. I wanted to go home because, regardless of the results, I knew I was going to get emotional. Good news and I would have cried tears of joy; bad news and I really would have cried and broken down badly I'm sure. Hey, like most men, I didn't want to show my emotions in the office. So, I got into my car and raced home.

As I walked into my place, out of habit I turned on the television for company. A ladies golf tournament was in progress. I sat down on the couch by the phone, waiting for Lisa's call...*Scared...worried, uptight. The phone rang and it was Lisa. She said, "Jerry, we cannot find the cancer anywhere except for one small spot, and we think that's likely scar tissue."*

As expected, when I hung up, I burst out balling with tears of joy! Relief. Joy! I didn't get a tissue. I got a towel...and needed every inch of it!

As I sat back down and tried to pull myself together, I began to focus on the television and the golf tournament.

At that moment, the sports announcer said, *"Folks, here's something we just have to show you. We shot this while we were on commercial break."* There on the screen, and consuming the whole screen, was a close-up shot of a beautiful hummingbird hovering over a flower! Well, I had to go and get another towel! Thank You, God...amazing love...awesome God!

Now you can think what you want, and I am sure some of you will. As far as I am concerned, God was sending me a note saying, *"You are going to be just fine and I will continue to watch over you." "Those were My footprints in the sand."* As for the 27 percent survival chance, well, the statisticians did not figure God into the equation. And I will carry this story to my grave, always believing God did in fact, send me a very personal message.

Take it one more step. I believe God sends us all messages. We just need to do a better job of recognizing them. We should always look for them…and keep looking for them.

Chapter 7

Visiting Old Friends

Shortly after finding out about having cancer, I went by to visit some old friends just to visit and share with them my bad news. Since we had moved away from Raleigh some years earlier, I had not seen them in a number of years. Larry and Pat Criminger and my family attended Millbrook Baptist Church together several years earlier and were in the same Sunday school class. That class was wonderful and was taught by one of the classist women I have ever met, Mrs. Gloria Norwood. To spend a Sunday morning in her class was like a breath of fresh air.

Pat and Larry were, and still are, thought of very highly by my entire family. I loved playing golf with Larry, and Scottie always enjoyed Pat's humor. One day Larry and I were playing golf and I was playing terribly. Larry shot a 73 that day and I believe I was more excited than he was. As I recall, he bogied the last hole to shoot that 73 and I enjoyed watching every moment of the day for him.

On my visit with Larry and Pat, I said I had cancer and the tears really began to flow…at least on my part. During our conversation, Pat said, *"We have a new pastor that I am sure you will like a lot. Why don't you go by and see him and the two of you can chat."* I called and set up an appointment and went by for my visit. The pastor's name was, the Right, Reverend, Dr. Robert Albritton, or as he would say, you can just call me Bob.

We immediately became friends and I must have gone through two or three boxes of his Kleenex. I did repay that debt of Kleenex a few days later. We eventually joined Millbrook Baptist and were all very happy at this church. We made friends that are friends to this day.

Later on in the process of my chemo sessions, Bob asked if I would like to give a testimony on Sunday to the congregation. He said to let everyone know what you are going through and the role Christ is playing in this whole situation. I told him I would.

I spent many restless nights trying to put together the correct words. I would wake up during the middle of the night and write down notes so I would not forget them in the morning. I prayed daily for Christ to help me with my words, I prayed until I sweated.

I called Bob one day and said I didn't know if I would be able to say everything I wanted to say in just ten minutes. His response was, *"Take as long as you like, but I'm leaving at 12:00 noon to go to lunch."* I took his lead and added a few more things to my notes.

The week before I was to give my testimony, Scottie and I had to be out of town and I really can't remember why. With us not being there for Sunday service, Bob had the opportunity to set me up for the greatest display of Christian love and support that I have ever seen in my life!

Giving my testimony that Sunday was probably one of the most difficult talks I have ever given. My goal was to get through it without crying. (Since I do cry at grand openings of 7-11 stores. My dear friend (Bill Thames) beat me however, he said he cried at the ground breaking of 7-11 stores) It was close on several occasions, but I didn't. Probably the toughest was while I was talking, I happened to look at my brother who had come over from Fayetteville, NC to hear the testimony, and he was boo-hooing pretty good, but somehow I held it back.

When I had finished, I told everyone thank you, and please keep me in their prayers. As I was walking off the pulpit, Bob stood up and said, "Wait a minute Jerry, there is something I need to tell you. He said everyone in the church loves you, but a lot of the people are upset that you are the only one in the church that gets to wear a baseball or golf hat to church each Sunday.
(To cover my somewhat bald head, from the chemo.)

But in spite of that, we all would like to show you how much we do love you. Just as he finished talking he reached around and came up with a baseball hat and put it on. Then the entire congregation reached down and picked up a hat and put it on. As I turned around towards the choir, everyone in the choir was wearing a hat. WOW, at that point, I lost it big time and the tears were bigger than elephant tears.

I left the pulpit and went into a little room to gather myself before going back into the sanctuary to take my place with Scottie. When I got seated, it was very obvious she had been crying. Scottie Wilson was a very strong woman and in all the years we had been married, I had only seen her cry a few times. I said to her, "Scottie, was I that good"…she just shook her head saying no and then it hit me, all that vanity. She was blown away, as I was, by what has to be the greatest displays of Christian love I have ever witnessed, everyone putting on a hat to show me how much they loved and cared for me. That special day will be embedded in my heart and mind for as long as I live.

Chapter 8

Cancer Again?

Diagnosed in 1996 with Stage 4 Lymphoma, Hodgkin's disease, I was pronounced cancer-free in 1997, or at least the cancer was in remission. After over 17 years later, I am still going strong.

In March 2012, I was diagnosed with cancer of the prostate gland. Prior to treatment in 2012, my PSA was 7.4; and my Gleason score was $3 + 3 = 6$ (A formula used to calculate the number of cancer cells in a biopsy.) The Gleason score is used to better guide a practitioner in making a decision about the next procedure.

I've told you about scary and about crying tears of joy. We were suddenly talking male anatomy…EF 4-tornado scary. A prostate cancer diagnosis demanded serious, serious research. Surgery and various related treatment procedures could result in horrible side effects. I, at this point in my life, just wanted to live a normal adult life.

God had compassion on me again. How I love Him. This time, He supernaturally sent someone into my sister Beverly's 360 beauty salon to talk about a treatment program called "Proton Therapy." It's a relatively non-invasive, target-specific treatment available now to most prostate cancer patients.

Continuing my pursuit to find the best possible direction to take for my treatment, I read a piece written by a friend (Dr. David Gilbert.) Dr. Gilbert also had prostate cancer at the time of his writing his piece, so you can rest assured, he did his homework. The title of his piece is called..."Sailing with Prostate Cancer." It contained a lot of factual material with a small dose of humor mixed in, which I enjoyed.

One comment he made in his piece I found particularly interesting...there are several ways to treat prostate cancer. In medicine, this usually means that one is not better than the other. An interesting comment since there are as many as double digit ways to treat prostate cancer.

His recommendation, (or at least, the one he seemed to favor) was the use of proton therapy because it was the least invasive means of treatment. (Age also plays a part in anyone's decision.)...Dr. Gilbert chose to use the normal form of radiation (locally) because he did not want to take the eight weeks off from his practice and travel to one of only a few locations that offer proton treatment. I had dinner the other night with him and his lovely wife, Gail. He is doing very well today, but still can't play golf worth a lick, so maybe he should have taken the time off for the proton treatment and for golf school in Florida! If Dave reads this book, he will know that I am only kidding here. I value his and Gail's friendship a great deal.

I wasted no time in making contact with the treatment center, talking with former patients, rearranging my life, relocating briefly to Florida, and taking on Cancer, Round two.

I have a friend who owns a place at beautiful Amelia Island, just about 30 minutes driving to the treatment center. He offered me his home...amazing how it all fell together. Blessed again! Do you think *Someone* was in charge and looking and taking care of me? I do!

Hoping to ward off loneliness while in Florida, I decided to keep in touch with friends and family by texting, calling, and emailing. My support group included Bill Kirby, Jr., friend, Putt-Putt golf star, and reporter and columnist for *The Fayetteville Observer*.

I think Bill Kirby was short on column inches when he agreed to run my journal under the paper's web site in 2012. He told me it was not a journal, but a blog...of course my next question was, "What is a Blog?"

 It sounded like something unclean to me. Regardless, he ran his blog which was my journal from Florida which I wrote each and every day for eight weeks.

During treatment for my second bout with cancer, I would entertain new friends, invite family and friends to come down, dine exquisitely, and often go to the golf course. Sounds like the ideal treatment for cancer to me, what do you think?

Oh, and every night I would write for the blog. My humor was still intact. My support group said they looked forward to the blog every day for many weeks. Writing the blog gave me something to look forward to during eight weeks of treatment far from home. It made the whole process more like a boondoggle than a nightmare. What a contrast to chemo.

God again blessed me! A year after treatment, in the summer of 2013, my PSA score was 0.06. I passed my first annual checkup for prostate cancer. I am currently leading a somewhat normal life, with no side effects from the 39 proton treatments. I might add here, normal is a little different for me.

Maybe the joke was on Bill. He was clueless at first about how his workload would increase…having to correct my long pages of spelling and grammatical errors. Well, he used it anyway. Not only did I come home healed; but also, I became a published author in the local newspaper.

Humor in the blog would supply my basic idea for a plot about the impact of attitude on health in **Cancer…A Blessing?** While other chapters set up the background and characters for the blog, I think the blog is the heart of this book. But other chapters show how my two ordeals with cancer affected me. For health's sake, Readers, I invite and gently encourage you to try a positive attitude for life.

Chapter 9

Cancer Is So Limited!

My story is somewhat unique in that I survived *cancer twice.* And those odds are not normal. I do understand that many cancer patients have been less fortunate than I.

God blesses us, but the devil steals, kills and destroys. **And nobody makes it through life without problems,** (Some are bigger than others.) For those who love and trust Him, God can work bad things into serving His purpose. We play a role in what happens in our lives, although most of us have a ways to go here....*I chose to fight!*

I would be remiss if I didn't share something I read while waiting to take chemo one day. Quoted below, the words molded my attitude in coping with cancer. They became my battle plan for successfully coping with a horrible disease. Even though the author is unknown, the words are so precious and priceless for me that I keep them in my Bible to this very day.

"Cancer is so limited...

It cannot cripple love
It cannot shatter hope
It cannot corrode faith
It cannot destroy peace
It cannot kill friendship
It cannot suppress memories
It cannot silence courage
It cannot invade a soul
It cannot steal eternal life
It cannot conquer the spirit

(Author Unknown)

I pray that each and every one of you use the above as your battle plan when you are informed of those three words..."You have cancer."

Chapter 10

How Can It Be A "Blessing"?

My story is somewhat unique in that I survived cancer twice. And those odds are not normal, especially with one of the bouts being stage 4!

My first bout with cancer was like a wake-up call from God. And I admit that in the middle of my crisis I saw cancer as a curse. Perhaps the second cancer was a reminder to keep my eyes on Jesus, to keep growing. I realized in hindsight that surviving cancer was actually a blessing for me – many blessings. I want others to be victorious like me. So, the writing of this book made me aware that cancer had brought positive, constructive changes that were blessings in my life.

Fighting cancer cracked opened the door to a better understanding of our role in our health and in being healed. The New Testament teaches us to believe God's promises in order to receive them. ("Just now leaving the station on this.") Jesus healed many during His ministry. And if a positive attitude impacts our own bodies, it probably can serve a role in lifting up others, influencing or helping them…like a cycle of giving and healing.

Because of cancer, I began to try to live life more fully, realizing how short this earthly life is. I want to make the most of every single day, even in retirement. Change can be a challenging and slow process for a senior, but I am working on it.

The cancer ordeals made me more thankful for all my blessing – and I don't mean just material blessings. I am much more aware of God's beauty in our natural world.

I used to ignore sunsets and flowers and hummingbirds. Not anymore. I see God's handiwork all around my yard. What an awesome Creator!

Because of cancer, I am thankful for my many support groups. Connecting with others is important. For me, that is family, friends, and my church family. There's plenty of research about how people can affect our emotional and physical health. In my experience, you need people in a health crisis. It is so important to surround ourselves with others who love the Lord, "Like-minded believers." Regularly attending church will not get us into heaven, but it can be a source of support to help us through our health trials.

My cancer ordeals have worked personal changes in me, changes that have impacted my goals and values. And these changes are still happening. I'm thinking they might be a part of God's plan, working something horrible into something really good. After all, I believe we are all WIP's… Works in Progress.

Surviving cancer positively impacted my relationship with my family. It is helping me to be a better listener, to be more loving, and to be more capable of hearing or seeing other people's needs. Agree or disagree, but I think it is moving my focus off of myself.

Surviving cancer made me more capable of serving God. For example, while I was sick, I was forced to surrender control to God, to submit to and depend on Him. James 4:7 tells us to submit to God, to draw near to Him and He will draw near to us. Maybe through the ordeal with cancer, God had a chance to reshape my heart and soul. My love and my relationship with Jesus grew stronger. Like many in the Bible, I'm not perfect...no, far from it. I know we are in a spiritual war and the devil attacks every day. But because of the illness, I realized the real Source of my strength. And because of the illness, I have learned how to submit to Jesus as the Lord of my life. I had to submit to serve and survive.

I also needed compassion to serve God and other people. Surviving cancer gave me compassion for cancer patients and their challenges. I realized I can be a blessing just with my presence, my sharing and my support. (And you can also) My skills with conversation improved, and I learned the power of humor. While volunteering at the Cancer Center here in Fayetteville, NC, I often chatted quietly with patients in the chemo room. Within minutes I could tell who would respond well to the chemo and who would not. The patients' attitudes were the driving force.

As a result of the ordeals with cancer, I had a strong desire to encourage others, to try to help by sharing my story. So, my book is intended to bless others through a record of words about experiences, my growth and some suggestions. I hope to show that, with the right tools, weapons and support, cancer doesn't have to be a death sentence.

Surviving cancer inspired me to do things for others, to volunteer to help people. For several years I headed up the support group at Snyder Memorial Baptist, a cancer support group. We had numerous speakers whose messages lifted us up and inspired us. And for eight years, I served as a volunteer at the Cancer Center of Cape Fear Valley Medical Center in Fayetteville, North Carolina. The Fayetteville Observer ran a column in 2012 about my treatments written by Bill Kirby. Tara Hinton, volunteer coordinator at the center, was quoted in it as saying, "Jerry has been a wonderful volunteer assisting patients and families." Even as a senior, I try to offer my help in the community.

Pastor John Cook, (COL., US Army {Ret}), senior pastor at Snyder Memorial Baptist Church, has been quoted as having said about me: "We affectionately call Jerry "Job", because of the many challenges he has faced and overcome in his life. He battled and beat cancer 17 years ago…He lost his precious wife, Scottie, unexpectedly…Any one of these events by itself could bring a man to his knees. Not only has he weathered these storms with his faith intact, but he has been an inspiration to all of us. He loves the Lord with all his heart, and he knows it is God's grace that has brought him safe thus far." John also said this past Sunday, something I have never heard, *"The opposite of fear is faith"*. Faith conquers fear, and quite frankly, you have to have it to go into battle with cancer.

Fighting cancer was both a physical and spiritual battle. Each of us has the responsibility to know and to believe promises in God's Word, to have faith, and to pray. Simply standing firm in faith requires prayer and belief in what the Bible says. To fight the devil and be a conqueror in Jesus Christ, we need to renew our minds by reading and understanding the Word. The Apostle Paul wrote in Hebrews 11:6, "But without faith it is impossible to please him: for he that cometh to God must believe that He is, and that He is a rewarder of them that diligently seek him." I believe that means God will bless us for believing in Him. We will be rewarded with eternal life.

As our Father, God wants a close relationship with us kids. Like any dad, God wants love and obedience. Being a dad myself, I like for my kids to stay in close touch, not to call only when they need something and always keep the line of communications open. I am so proud of my kids for conforming to this and have always respected the line of communication they both had with their mother. Of course, she was an incredible communicator.

Do you need answers? Take time to get to know the Heavenly Father. As much as you are physically and mentally able, draw closer to God. That comes from Bible reading and prayer. The Bible is God's love letter to us. Proverbs 8:17 says, "I love them that love me; and those that seek me early shall find me." On a daily basis I live life trying to do what I feel is God's will. Getting close to God helps. It can turn your attitude into your secret weapon. Hey, it even might make you a better person. Perfect, NO, but a better person none the less.

A friend said to me recently, "I'm sure God has way bigger plans for you, yet to be done on this earth." I am confident of that fact – because of how cancer brought changes into my life.

For anyone just diagnosed with cancer, I suggest not sticking your head in the sand, moping around, saying *"Oh, woe is me."* On the other hand, I suggest not trying to beat it by yourself. Try turning it all over to God…"Casting all your care upon Him, for he cares for you." (I Peter 5:7) And put forward your best attitude.

We all will face trials in life. Through my story, I hope others will renew their minds and learn to lean on God. Oh, and those footprints in the sand belong to the carpenter. He promised to help us. Why not let Him help carry you through those trials?

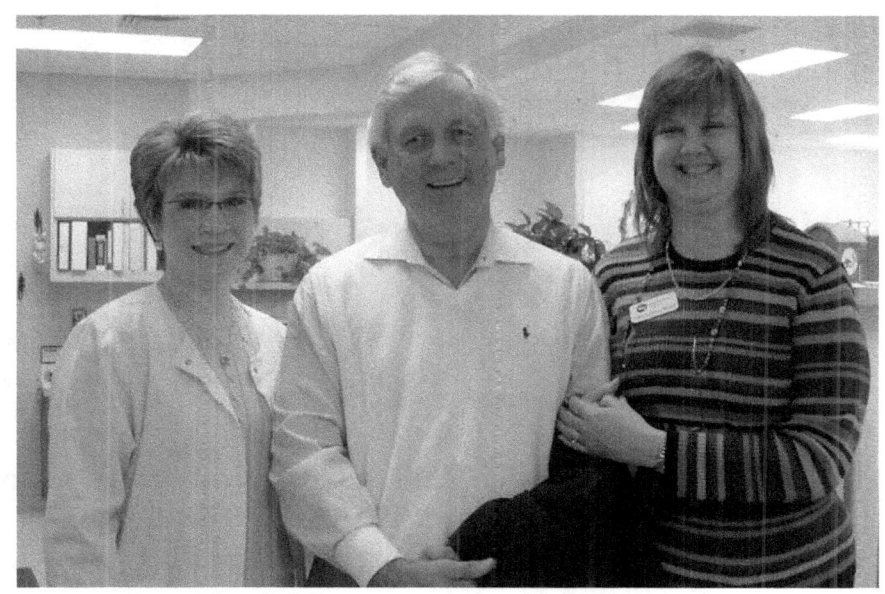

Jennifer & Lisa on a visit a few years ago

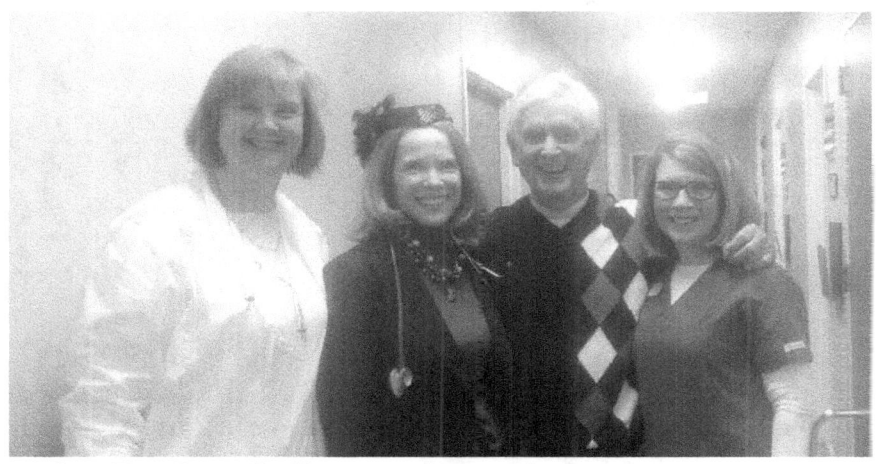

Lisa, Dr. Campbell, me and Jennifer on a very recent visit

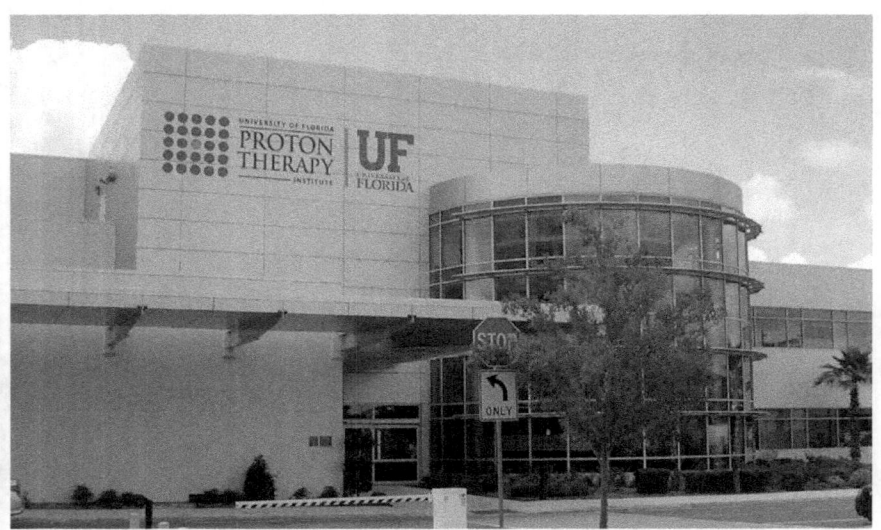

University of Florida Proton Treatment Center,
Jacksonville, Fla.

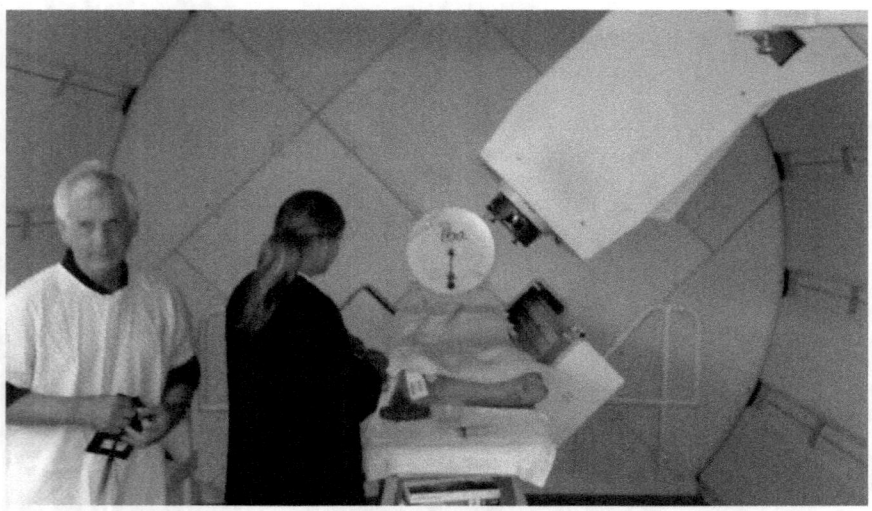

The *"Gantry"* where the treatments were administered

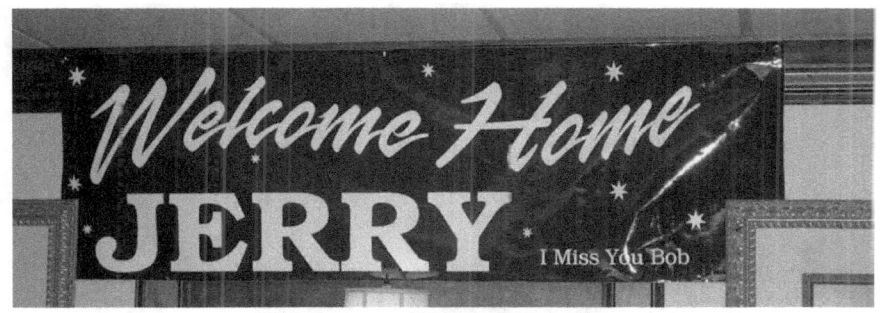

"Welcome Home Sign"

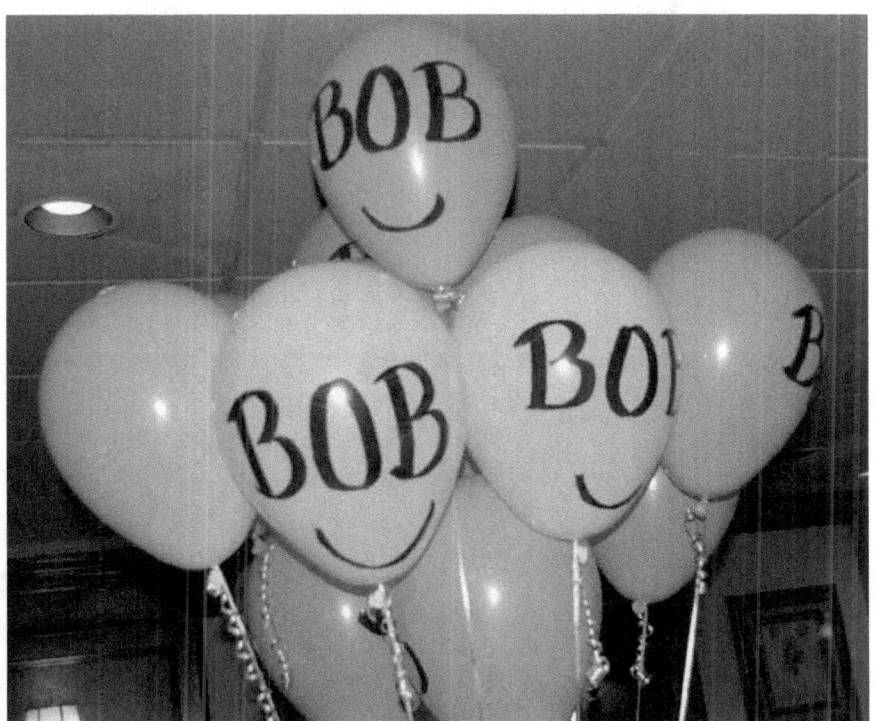

My Friend "BOB"! from Florida. You will find out more about him later on!

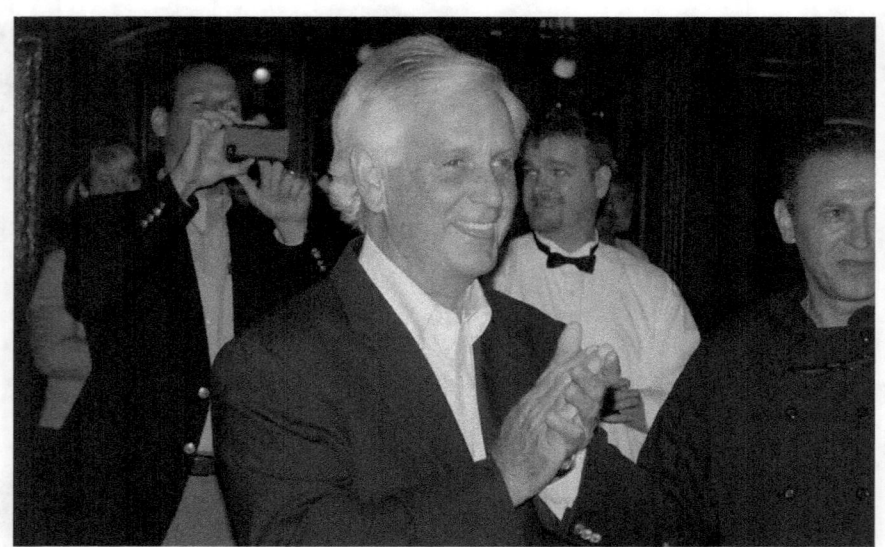

Arriving and applauding everyone that attended
the welcome home party

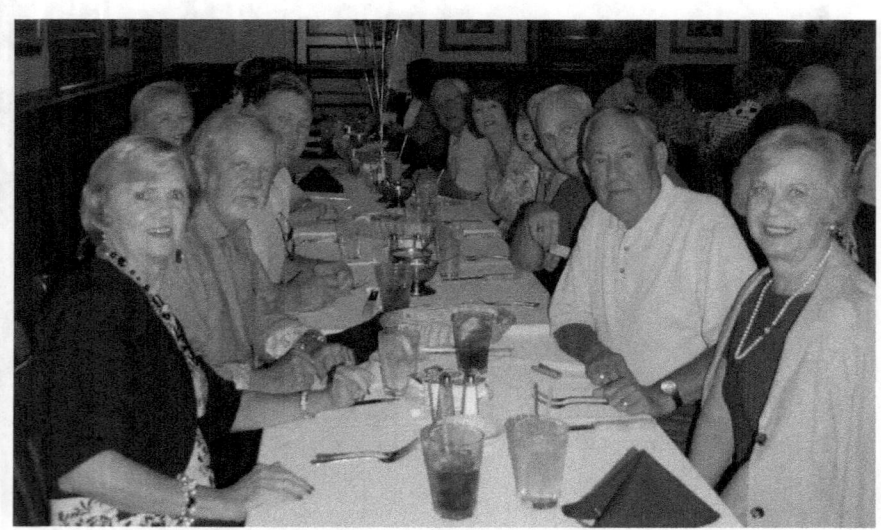

Some of the guests, almost 100 attended!

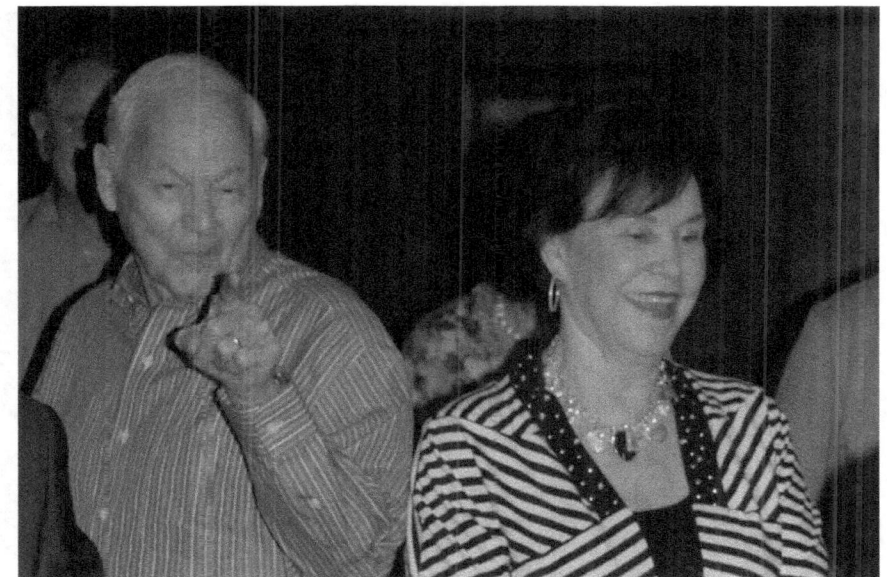

"Got you", my dear friend Stan and his wife Faye Griffin

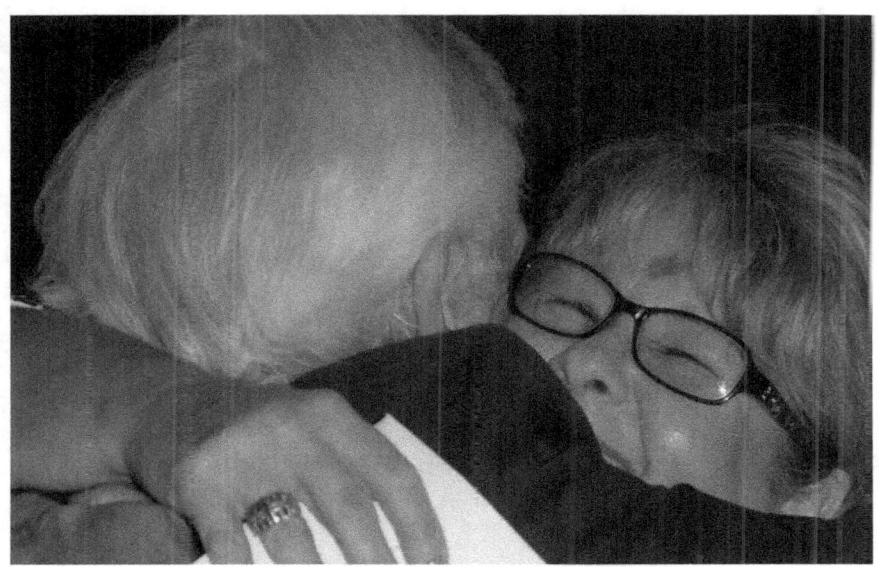

Sister, Beverly welcoming me home

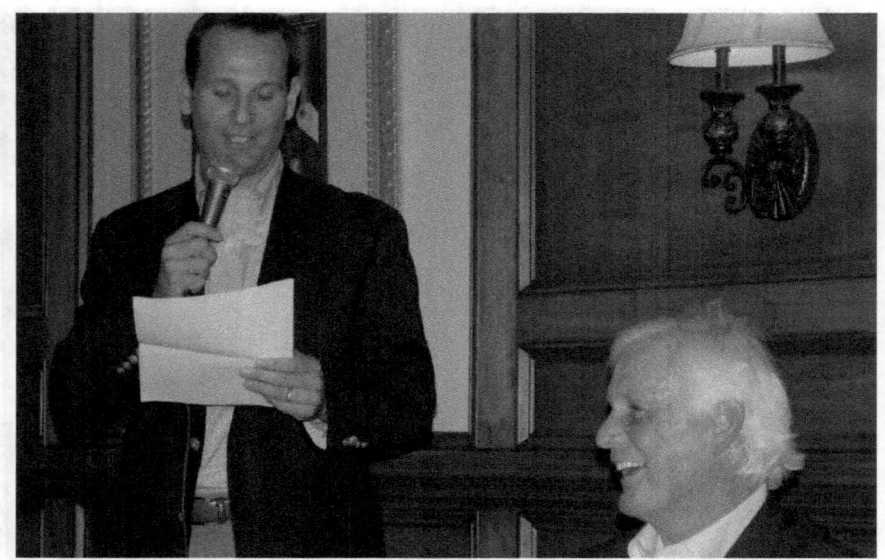

My Son giving a little talk and trying to be funny…he was!

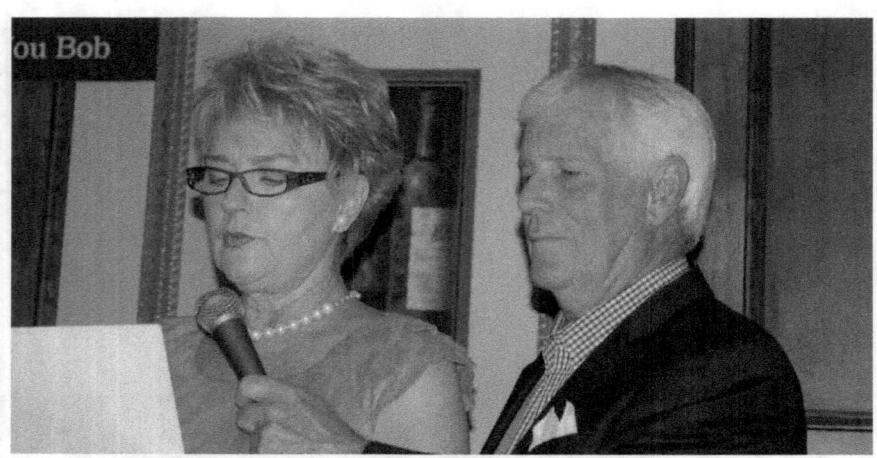

Gary and Brenda on a more serious note

My son, Keith with his wife, Sherie-Beth, with Grace
and Luke

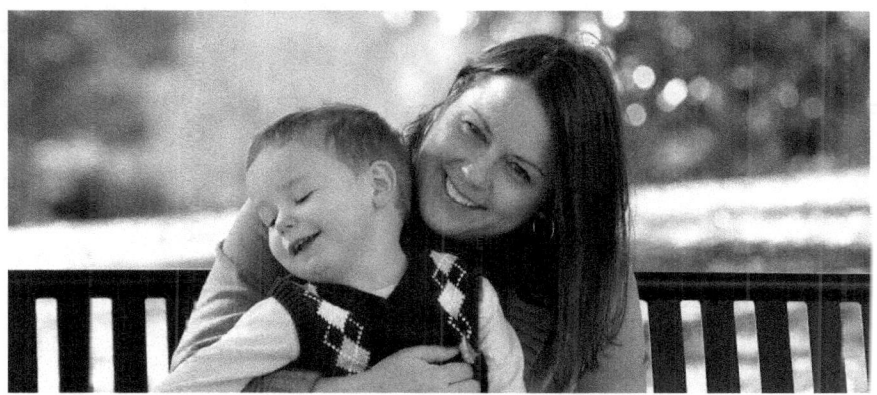

My daughter, Kim, and her precious son, Caden

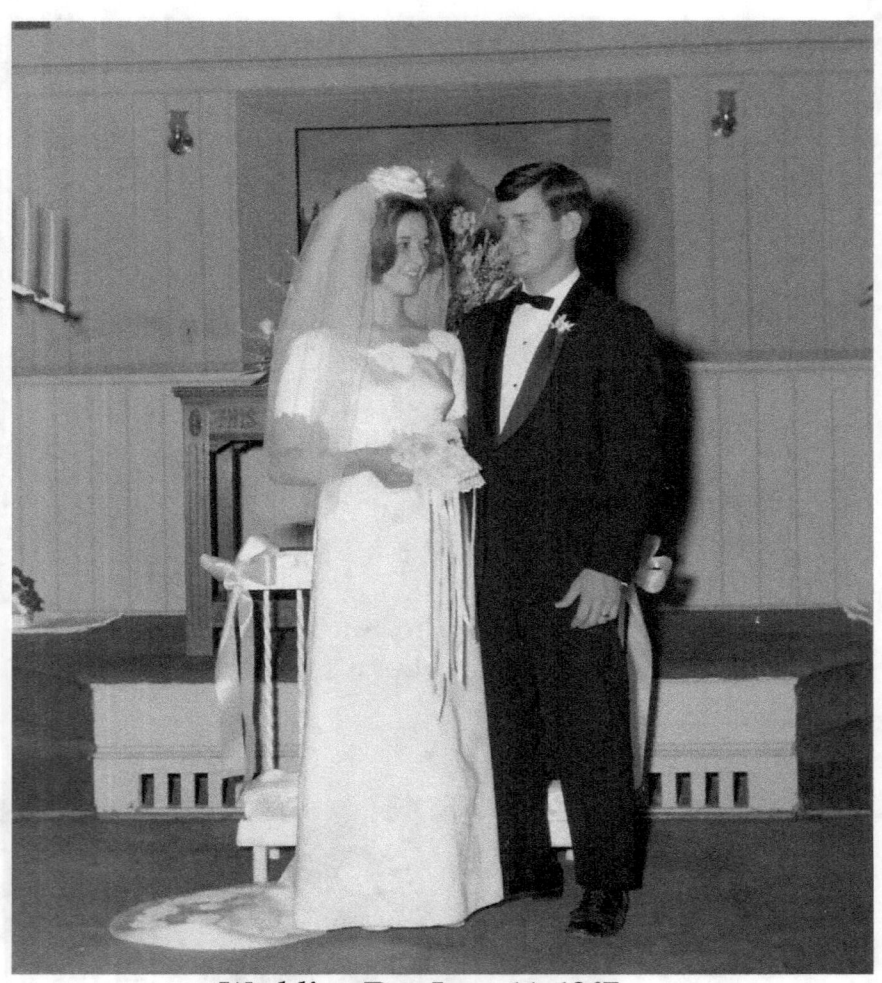

Wedding Day June 11, 1967

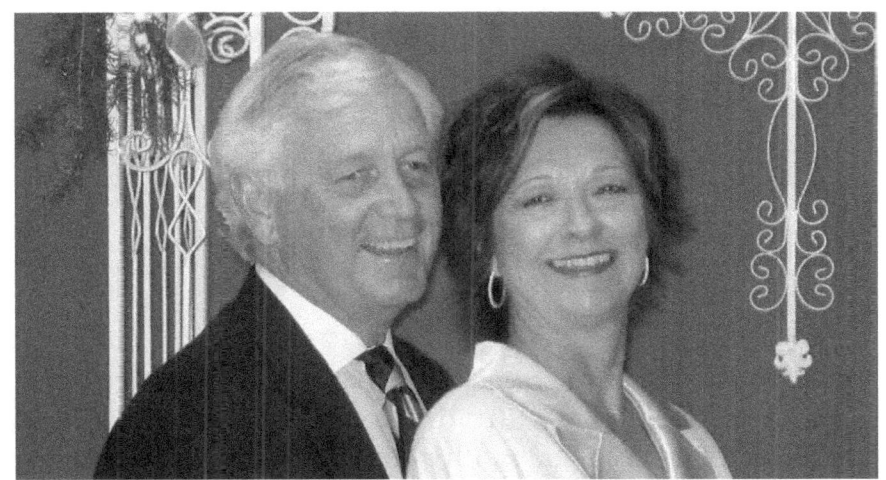

40th Wedding Anniversary (Renewing Vows)

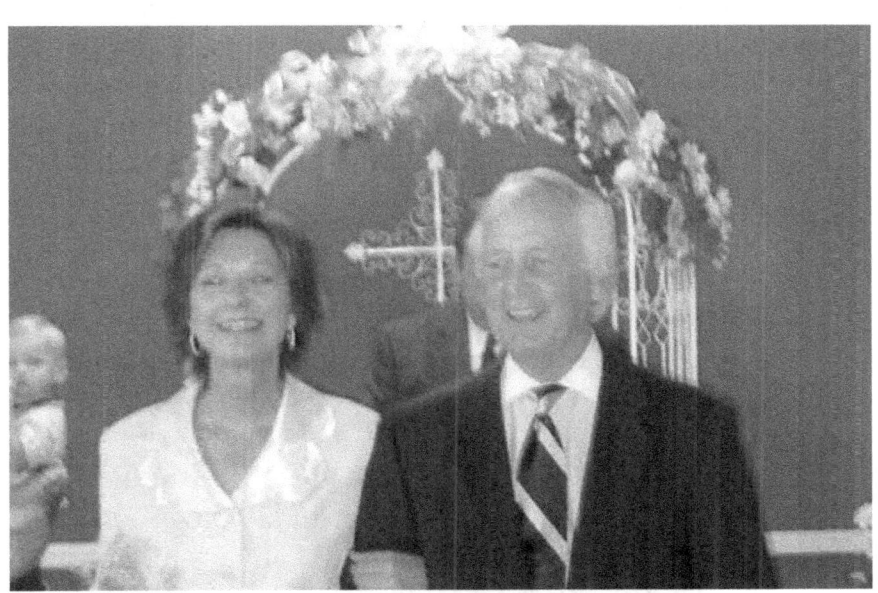

40th Wedding Anniversary

Explanation....

A little insight…the remaining chapters will take you off on another journey with a different twist…same evil character (cancer), but with a different name.

I was diagnosed with prostate cancer in 2012. After much research and investigation of possible treatments, I decided on Proton Therapy in Jacksonville, Florida. This treatment was chosen because it was far less invasive with virtually no side effects. It definitely was not an easy decision, but to this day, I feel like I made the right one. In fact, there is no doubt in my mind.

While in Florida for treatment, I decided to record my activities each day so that I might have something to reflect back on when finished…I called it a journal…later to be informed I was wrong, it should have been called a blog.

Bill Kirby (Writer for The Fayetteville Observer, local newspaper) was kind enough to print my blog each day. A few said they enjoyed it, one said, I always thought you were a nut, this blog confirms it! And that person knows who he is…my friend.

The remaining chapters are as they appeared in the newspaper each day. (Being used with permission from the paper). I ask the reader to keep in mind, the blog was not written as a book and was never intended to be one. Because of that, you can expect to see a very liberal use of literary license. Keep in mind, it was written to be informative, but for fun and enjoyment...please enjoy.

Chapter 11

A Journey With Me

Week One

<u>June 17, 2012 (Sunday)</u> **Two types of men**

Someone told me once; there are two types of men...men that have prostate cancer, and men that are going to get prostate cancer. Although prostate cancer is not what I had to deal with 17 years ago, (Lymphoma (Hodgkin) stage 4 cancer) it is cancer. God's grace (and many prayers from friends and family) got me through that horrible experience 17 years ago, and He will get me through this as well, there is no doubt in my mind.

The following is a day by day experience of my trip to Jacksonville Fla., to participate in the little know Proton Therapy. First and foremost, I feel very confident that I have chosen the best treatment for my issue. I am also grateful beyond measure for the generosity of a friend in Christ that has so generously let me stay in his beautiful place on Amelia Island. It is beautiful and decorated to the nines. The toilet seats even closed automatically....cool. I almost feel guilty, feeling like I'm on some type of vacation. The vacation will start tomorrow.

 Having been through a simulation of the treatment on an earlier visit to Florida, it's not going to be a vacation, but far easier that the numerous times I had to take chemo and give myself shots daily to build up my white count during my previous treatment for cancer. Being so vain, I'm also thankful that during this type of treatment, I don't lose any of my hair....not very pretty without hair!

All set and ready to go. Car is packed with far too many clothes, now all I have to do is set the alarm system and I'm on my way. Oh no, the alarm system which was recently updated and installed with monitoring does not work.

What will I do? I called the Holmes Electric people and they were very swift in taking care of my problem. The technician arrived within 15 or 20 minutes and took care of my problem and now I was on my way.

I had a book on tape that my son had given me for Father's day and had planned on listening to it on the way to Florida. The book is called "Calico Joe" by John Grisham. It's about a baseball experience and one that I was really looking forward to helping me get through 6 and a half hours of driving. (Not to mention my interest in baseball). Well I was really enjoying the book when I found myself asleep driving down the middle of the road....scary. Well, what was I going to do? I had five plus more hours of driving and for some reason, could not stay awake. Stopped at a 7-11 store and bought a 5 hour pick me up drink. After all, if Jim Furyck can take it to play golf, why couldn't I use it to help me drive without falling asleep. It worked: I was able to continue my trip to Fla., without any other issues....well almost. I was so alert that I forgot what the speed limit was and got a ticket.

I was so nervous, which is totally unlike me. I guess it was due to the fact that I have not had a ticket in years...many years. On top of that, this was the first time

I have been stopped since I now have a concealed weapon permit and carry a Smith and Wesson 38 in the car with me on trips. I put both hands on the steering wheel and told the officer I had a loaded 38 in my console and felt like Barney with his one bullet...I could hardly talk. He really didn't care to hear about my weapon, but was more interested in collecting a little more revenue for the state of Georgia. I was less than three miles from the Florida border....a speed trap maybe?

Arrived safely, but worn out from the trip and my grandson's 1st birthday party the day before, which turned out great. I put a $50 minimum on gifts and he made out well. Watched a little of the US Open and then to bed. Figured I would find out who won in the morning.

June 18, 2012 (Monday) **Now, Mr. Wilson, are you Ready?**

Big day today, first treatment at 2:20 in the afternoon. Spent most of the morning just relaxing. Read a little about how Tom Watkins hits a golf ball....swing back and shake hands, swing forward and shake hands.

The golf swing is just that simple. I searched the internet a little. Checked email (how did we live without it) and had some nice comments from friends and relatives wishing me well. Went out to the pool for a bit, but I was the only one there, must be out of season here in Florida.

Finally, time to head to the treatment center. Met with my own special nurse, Barbara to review some vitals. They haven't changed a bit, but they always ask you what meds you are on. I also told her that I doubt they would change anytime in the near future since I was going to be here until sometime in August. She asked me a bunch of other questions, but I can't type them here as they were all personal. For example, how many times do I get up during the night to go to the bathroom? I lied and told her....never, but finally told her the truth since I think that's important information for them to know. Met with the doctor for about 5 minutes, I wonder how much he made for that 5 minutes....I should have been a doctor.

Treatment time....they took me in a room that looked something like it came from star wars (It's called the gantry). Machines and gadgets everywhere, and I mean big machines! Checked to see if my bladder was full...that's important (When it's full, it keeps the prostate stationary). Now it's time for the balloon (Bob, they call it). They put that balloon where the sun doesn't shine and fill it up with saline to keep the prostate stationary....that was fun. Oh, the balloon does not have a happy face on it. Now, Mr. Wilson, are you ready, yes I replied and the treatment took all of about a minute and a half. Technology....wow has it changed.

Home now; it's almost 8:30, close to my bed time. I will report in tomorrow...**Good night everyone.**

June 19, 2012 (Tuesday) **This is God**

Well, the first day may have taken its toll on me; I did not wake up until 9 am. It was probably a combination of the drive down, first treatment and the Melatonin....You think! Not sure what I'm going to do today, probably go for a walk on the beach and get a little sun, after all I do want to come back to Fayetteville cured of cancer, tall, dark and handsome.

Well, cured of cancer will be fine. My treatment time today is 4:30. My daughter Kim sent me a saying several years ago that I will always remember..."This is God. I

79

will be handling all your problems today. I don't need your help". Well I sure wish he would make that balloon a little smaller!

Just got back from a walk to the beach...it takes about 5 minutes to get to the beach. God's construction of this earth continues to amaze me...the beauty is breathtaking. Passed one of the golf courses, The Links I believe, what a beautiful hole I saw. The buildings, homes and condos are beyond my debt of reality....millions of dollars. One of the areas here reminds me of Magnolia Lane at Augusta Ga., the Masters. The beautiful trees engulf the road and make it look like a tunnel.

While on the phone with Greg C. he asked for some information that I had in the car. I told him I would call him right back with that information. I opened the front door and just as it closed realized the key was in side. Yes, I had locked myself out of the house! No shoes, no wallet, no phone, but most important, no key!!!!! I guess I was lucky to have had my pants on. I walked over to the tennis courts and a lady that was there while her son was taking a lesson let me use her phone. I called Gary and he got in touch with the owner who was on the golf course. My friend called the real estate office and they brought me another key. Don't you just love old people? At that point I was able to make my second appointment with the balloon. Joked some with the nurses that inserted it (Can't repeat what I said to them here) and the treatment from that point went well. Stopped at Harris Teeter on the way home and picked up some grouper and slaw for dinner and that pretty much ended the day.

Good night everyone.

June 20, 2012 (Wednesday) **New Friends**

Having a cup of coffee as treatment today is 8pm this

evening. I guess that kind of makes it a date. But what the heck, two down and only 37 left....piece of cake.

Made two new friends today. While cleaning off the deck, and looking for a hose to wash it down I met two of the cleaning staff....Carla and Joanne. They were very delightful & helpful, but we found no hose, but two new friends none the less.

Well the treatment center called and had an earlier opening which I took at 4:40. Met a gentleman from Tampa (Tim) and enjoyed my conversation with him. He is seven days ahead of me. We had some laughs talking about the balloon, but it's really not funny. You folks need to pray until you sweat to get the enormous size of this balloon down. By the way, I learned today that the balloon has a nickname....it's called BOB. In the future I will refer to the balloon as BOB. The treatment went well and I continue to feel so blessed to have chosen this type of treatment...God is so good. As I left the center today they told me my treatment tomorrow will be at 7:45 pm, hope they call me tomorrow also with an earlier time.

Interesting dinner tonight, half a bag of Cheetos and some grapes. Is that a balanced meal or what?

Good news.....I went all day and did not lock myself out of the house!!!!

Good night everyone.

June 21, 2012 (Thursday) I **Trust in God**
Today, my appointment was scheduled for 7:45 pm, but they just called and asked if I could come in at noon....sounds good to me.

How did I hear about this Proton Therapy? Good question? Duke will not tell you about it, Chapel Hill either, and surprisingly most of the doctors are unaware of it. So, after all my research, here's how it happened.

My sister who owns 360 Beauty Salon was doing this ladies hair who works at a dentist office. She had just finished cleaning someone's teeth that had told her about this treatment, because he had just been through it. Beverly called me and I was able to get in touch with David Kirkpatrick and he filled me in. I called the Proton Center and asked for information. After reviewing the material, and calling some of the 350 names they sent me as references, I decided this was it. One person I called was taking a nap and I spoke with his wife. Her comment was she thanked God for allowing this type of treatment to be discovered. That was it for me. As my friend says, I trust in God, I believe he knows what he is doing....makes perfectly good sense to me. Oh, what were my other options?

- Watch it and see if it gets any worse
- Radical Surgery
- Robotic Surgery
- Freeze it (brr, brr)
- Radiation
- Seeds
- Special Seeds done in Atlanta
- Another type Seed
- HIFU, which is done outside the country.
- I'm sure I'm overlooking one or two.
1. OK, it's your decision, which one do you want???????

Today my friend David will be here in town for his one year checkup and hopefully we will be able to meet and chat. I've never met him in person and look forward to meeting him.

On the way home from treatment I stopped at the

Fernandina Beach Golf Club. Went in and introduced myself to the Pro....Carl, and I went out and hit a big bag of balls. I hope the treatment is working on my cancer, hasn't done a thing for my golf swing, but after all, I am half of the winning team for the Highland Country Club Member Guest. Ok, Gary played very well....but I helped a little!!!!!!

Got an email earlier from my friend Susan and she suggested I get some exercise while I'm here. After thinking about it I went out and bought a speedo to swim and do laps in the pool. When I showed up at the pool in my speedo, all the women and children left screaming and crying....maybe I picked the wrong color. I'm going to take it back tomorrow and get a white one.....not!!!!! Tomorrow being Friday will be my last day of treatment this week. Can't wait for the weekend and two days off. Weather permitting, I hope to play some golf and explore the Island.

Good night everyone.

<u>June 22, 2012 (Friday)</u> **Small Children**

Treatment today is scheduled for 7:15 tonight. Great way to start the weekend don't you think? Really, I'm just thankful the first week is almost over.

Although it has not been a bad week at all, it has taken an adjustment to being completely alone in a strange (but beautiful) area. Right now my two best friends are the receptionist....Dina & Terry. I call them Twiddle Dee and Twiddle Dumb....they call me Lockout....wonder why? Yes, I did share with them my earlier experience in the week when I locked myself out of the condo!

Do miss having breakfast with the president of the Mexican Mafia. He is always there for breakfast and is teaching me how to speak Spanish better.....which is difficult, since he doesn't speak a word of English. And all the other old f—t's, it's a great way to start the day.

Every once in a while, I will start to feel sorry for myself, but I get over it in a second when I see all the small children, from all over the world, that are here for some type of cancer treatment. I've met people from England and Scotland. More often than not, their treatment is for a much more severe cancer than mind!

Started to do some clothes washing this morning. My washer and dryer are very modern which I purchased some 20 plus years ago from Sears. Before starting here I had to google engineering degree, and I haven't even tried the dryer yet. I did look outside for a clothes line, but none was to be found....can you imagine in such a nice place there is no clothes line, oh well, no clothes pins either.

Well, they have done it again. The Proton Center just called and changed my time to 1pm. Let me go, got to jump into the shower. I always like to look my best for BOB!

What's for dinner? Decided to drive down the beach and eat at a place called the Surf. It was recommended by some people at the treatment center. Fried Shrimp, yummy. They had a fellow singing and playing the guitar...he was pretty good. He asked if I'd like to join him for a few songs, but I declined....was more interested in the shrimp. The strange thing to me as I drove down the coast line, none of the homes on the ocean front or a street back were built on poles. Everything was built, almost like on a concrete slab. What's that all about?
I just learned a dear friend lost his wife today and she was quiet the lady. I personally know and feel his pain and emptiness.

My heart goes out to him. She will be missed and my thoughts and prayers go out to my friend and his entire family. I know the wonderful Sunday school class is supporting him well. They sure did for me.

Good night everyone.

<u>June 23, 2012 (Saturday)</u> **Sandy Bottoms**

What a beautiful day so far, not a cloud in the sky. Started the day with a walk on the beach, surprised, not that many people. Came back to the pool and swam 40 laps for my daily exercise.....oops, sorry, that's a typo, only swam four laps, it's a small pool. But all kidding aside, it's great exercise, I believe you use every muscle in your body...hope I can do it every day and come home really buff, whatever that is?

Had lunch today at the Marehe Burette Deli. It was delicious, and I had the best tea I've ever had in my life. It's made out on the west coast, I believe, and it's called Pete's. Someone told me they made coffee also. I wish my friend and sister in law had been with me. Lee is a very special lady that I love dearly. Lee, they even had grey poupon, how about that. Lee we would have laughed our fannies off....I thought of you a lot while having lunch....Please tell Bobby and Denise I said hello. Denise, how is our place at Kure Beach doing? Bobby, you catching any flounder?

Went to hit golf balls after lunch at Amelia River Golf Club. They have an excellent driving range and I look forward to playing their course. Met a couple, Jim & Gayle on the range and they were very nice. Both retired and moved down here about 5 years ago. Jim was a Navy Pilot and a real gentleman. They have both just taken up the game....Oh well; it's not a perfect world, is it? They probably play like those Cook twins!!!!!

Has anyone every lost their cell phone? Well I misplaced
mine today and looked everywhere for it. Too bad I
didn't have a land line to call it to help me look for it.
You know you're getting old when you even look in the
refrigerator for it....and I did. Finally found out why it
was not in the house...it was in the car right where I left
it...oh well!!

Had dinner tonight at a place the treatment center people
recommended, called Sandy Bottoms. It was right on the
beach and you could even sit on the beach and be served.
They also had a singer performing, not sure what type of
music it was, but the guy had a great voice and I enjoyed
listening. I was more interested in his girlfriend, but for
some reason, she showed no interest in me.....do you
think it was the age difference...had to be! Maybe even
the grey hair.

Back home now and its almost 9:30. Wow, I have stayed
up half the night as my mother used to say.

Good night everyone.

Chapter 12

A Journey With Me

Week 2

<u>June 24 2012 (The Lord's Day)</u> **Snyder Choir**

Attended Amelia Baptist Church this morning and glad I did. The pastor Dr. Neil Helton was good (not as good as John Cook, but good. John asked me to say something nice about him in my journal if I got the chance!) and I enjoyed his sermon very much. When it was time for the choir to sing, about twenty some people just came out of the congregation and formed the choir. I thought to myself, how good could this be? (Shame on me) They were awesome!! They sang a song called "Written in Red" and it actually gave me chills. Reminded me of Scottie, and what she used to say about the Snyder Choir, she would say "the Snyder choir makes me sick and gives me the flu, because every time they sing, I get chills". I agree with her, we are so blessed to have so many musically talented people, and a wonderful pastor to boot. Snyder has definitely been blessed.

Had a great lunch. Cooked the left over grouper in lemon and butter and made a sandwich with cold slaw....it was yummy. Pretty much spent the day watching the golf tournament because of the rain.

This storm that's acting up in the gulf coast has created

some very rainy weather, but they are expecting it to clear up by Tuesday or Wednesday.
After all, they are correct 50% of the time. Also did some ironing...yes ironing? Not anything big, t-shirts, shorts etc. I even ironed a few paper napkins...you never know when someone might stop by and you always want to put your best foot forward. I can remember when my mother (Mrs. Barnhill) used to iron everything, including sheets, pillow cases and even our underwear.

As she said, you never know when you might have a wreck and have to go to the doctor or hospital. You sure don't want to go with dirty underwear for everyone to see!

Going to get a salad for dinner, watch 60 minutes and Sunday night baseball and call it a day. Yes I'm already getting excited meeting up with BOB tomorrow. I know he has missed me over the weekend.

Good night everyone.

June 25, 2012 (Monday) **An Olympic Beauty**

Monday morning and Amelia Island has survived the storm. Basically just a tropical storm Debby. Raining pretty heavy, with some flooding in Jacksonville, Fla., but things are looking up for the rest of the week. Well almost, there is that little appointment with BOB. Scheduled for my treatment appointment today at 6:30 this evening. Well what do you know; the center just called and have an opening at 1:50 so I'm heading out for Jacksonville. Things went well; I hope the rest of my treatments go as well. Just think I only have 33 more left.

I drove by Amelia River Golf Club to hit some balls and help pass the time and they were closed. They must have had some flooding from the Tropical Storm Debby.

These weather people don't even know how to spell, we all know its spelled Debbie....what were they thinking, but as I said earlier in this journal, they are only right 50% of the time. They missed this one.

Had a late lunch/dinner and met a couple from South Carolina. Hate that the Gamecocks did not win last night (College World Series). I'm sure my friend Ronnie Collins along with many others are disappointed, but 2 out of 3 is not a bad batting average.

Dinner time, let's see, where am I going for dinner. At lunch today they recommended Baxter's, so why not. So off to Baxter's I go. Only a few people there when I arrive so I go to the social area. Wasn't really hungry, so watched the people coming and going. Met a couple from upstate NY, and enjoyed their company. (Jim and Jane Beimer)

Another fellow joined them, Ethan, and talked with them about living in upstate NY for a couple of years. As it turns out, Ethan was a member of the TPC course at Sawgrass for 10 years so we discussed the course and #17 (A beautiful but dangerous par three) for quite a while. He also said he could get me on any course worthwhile in the area. I have his phone number, so we will see about that whenever this rain gets out of here.

Met another gentleman who was telling me his wife was going through chemo now for Lymphoma; I didn't ask him what stage she was in. I did however; tell him about Julia and how she had beaten it twice. Julia is also a great inspiration to many at the cancer center, as well as, all over Fayetteville.

All of a sudden this beautiful lady came through the front door with her husband. Not only was she beautiful, but had class written all over her. Ethan said, do you know who that woman is? Of course I didn't know so he told me. She is Mrs. Barbara Ann Scott (King), gold medalist in the 1948 Olympics for Canada. (She was an ice skater) WOW, I was more than impressed. She was a woman of grace, beauty, charm and elegance. I can just see her accepting the gold now.

When I got home I sat down at my laptop to look for emails and saw I had one from the couple I met during dinner tonight. (Jim & Jane) They told me how nice it was to meet me, and when they get back from upstate NY in a few weeks, he would take me out to Long Point Golf Course, one of the really nice ones here on the Island. WOW, it's almost 9:30,

Good night everyone.

<u>June 26, 2012 (Tuesday)</u> **The Mexican Mafia Called**

What a pleasant surprise this morning. Gary was at Lindy's, the breakfast place for champions and I got to speak to a lot of Champs. Charles, Uncle Bob, Bill J., Jimmy, Ron and Sue, Jr., and of course the Mexican Grand emperor of the Mexican mafia, Al.....nice surprise! Hope I didn't leave anyone off the above list, but you know how we old people are!

Rain, rain, rain, Jacksonville is expecting almost 10 inches of rain today. I will probably have to go in for my appointment by boat....not a bad idea! I've acquired several nicknames over the years...Dr. Wilson, Senator Wilson and a few I can't mention, but yesterday I changed it to <u>Noah</u>. I'm starting to build a boat this afternoon, but I believe I'm going to leave the animals off!

Had dinner at Baxter's last night. They make a great steak sandwich and it was delicious. My new friend

Ethan was there again last night also, so I joined him for dinner. In our conversation, I can't even remember all the places he has homes. He spends most of his time here on the plantation because his son lives here also. Also saw the Gold Medal winner again last night. I'm not sure how old she is (I'm guessing 85 or so) but she still looks like a tiny Barbie doll. Ethan reminded me he could get me on any course I wanted and specifically mentioned Long Point. I believe, that's one of the better courses here.....really looking forward to it, a lot of marsh on it, hope I brought enough golf balls.

Well it's late now, almost 10 pm.....**Good night everyone.**

June 27, 2012 (Wednesday) **University Club**

The next few lines or paragraphs have nothing to do with my journey against cancer, but rather some nice thoughts I had this morning that I wanted to reflect on. First, my daughter had a good day yesterday and received what we were praying for...what an awesome God. Secondly, my son and daughter in law gave me a Tassimo coffee maker. It's one of those fancy machines that makes one cup of coffee at a time. I brought it with me here and am continuing to enjoy it here. Scottie would have laughed at it....she drank so much coffee in the morning. Third, my devotional book given to me last Christmas by a dear friend (Jesus Calling, by Sarah Young). My new year's desire was to read it every day, along with the scripture it recommended. For the most part, I've read it every day and really feel like my life has been enriched by doing so. On top of that, one of my Sunday School Teachers uses the same devotional book. The more I can be like Becky, I feel the better off I will be, she is wonderful and has a true gift for teaching, along with many other talents. Our Sunday school class has been blessed with many talented instructors.

Now back to business. My appointment today is 4:30, followed by a doctor's appointment. I guess he feels like he needs a little more money, so he wants to see me to tell me how good I'm doing.

(Hope he doesn't ask me how I'm doing with BOB) After the doctor's appointment I'm going to dinner at the University Club. All patients are automatic members while we are here and it is first class on first class, no duct tape there Bobby Bryan. It's on the 28 floor and overlooks the entire city of Jacksonville, can't wait. (I also believe it turns while you are having dinner, giving you the entire view of this beautiful city).

University Club....WOW, WOW. It doesn't revolve as I thought, but it is on the 28th floor and overlooks the St. Johns River. The night was beautiful and the view was breathtaking. When it's dark, the city lights magnify on the River, making it even more beautiful. For dinner I had a small filet cooked medium rare and it was perfect. My beautiful friend had Shank of Lamb and said it was absolutely wonderful; it was so tender you could cut that shank with a fork. I told them I played golf, and I'm not ordering anything with the name Shank in it. It could be contagious....you just never know.

Oh, just as a side note, my doctor, Dr. Nichols said I was doing fine....!!

Good night everyone.

June 28, 2012 (Thursday) **My Friend, Frank Upchurch**
Appointment today was at 9:30 went well, and then off to St Augustine and the World Golf Hall of Fame. Enjoyed it very much, what a beautiful place. Got to hit one ball onto an Island green to win a poster of the latest inductees into the Hall of Fame. It was only a 132 yard hole. The prevailing winds were horrible, I didn't take

into consideration the earth's rotation, and worst of all, the dew point number was out of sight.....yes, and I missed the green!!! The beautiful lady that hit right after me must have worked for the weather station, and had all the important facts, she hit the green...! They gave her the inductee's poster and I begged her for it.....what a nice weather women, she gave it to me!! I did buy a killer hat while I was there and can't wait to get home and show it off.....

Heard from my buddy Frank Upchurch via email and he has a family friend here on the Island that he said I should stop by and see. Stopped by his store and they told me he would not be on the Island until Saturday. Will definitely go back. Anyone that has Frank Upchurch as a friend has got to be a quality act....Frank sure is! What an inspiration to everyone that knows him.

Well it's about 4:30 and seems like nap time to me.

Went back to Baxter's again tonight...and yes Mrs. Canadian Gold Medal winner was there again tonight. They must not have a stove in their home...you think? Had two of my favorite things for dinner. Fried green tomatoes with shrimp to get started, and Steak Diane for dinner...yummy, yummy, yummy.

Well, it's off to bed, have to meet with BOB in the morning at 7:20 (what a way to start your day), and then going to play golf at the Amelia River Golf Club.

Gary and Brenda are coming tomorrow. Really looking forward to their company.

Good night everyone.

June 29, 2012 (Friday) **Coconut Cream Pie!**
Another week over and here comes the weekend. I will

not miss BOB at all, sorry BOB, I'll see you Monday at 7:15 am. Got up at 5:30 because I had a treatment at 7:15 and what a view and pleasant drive down A1A....lots of water and beautiful views. I was back home in no time and got ready for my first day of golf here with my friend. We played Amelia River Golf Club...it was nice....#17 was set up a little like #17 at TPC Sawgrass, where they play the players championship. Thought about playing there once while I'm here and ask the people at the Proton Center if I could. They said yes, and it was off season now and I could play there for only $175 green fees.....I think not. Only place I would pay that is the Augusta National.....where they play the Masters Did a little cleaning for Gary and Brenda, rested, and oh yes, a little nap for the day. Gary and Brenda got here about 7:30 and we went to the Surf for dinner....it was very good. During dinner we planned our time while they are here and it looks like all we are going to do is eat.

Got home from dinner and opened my care package from home. Beverly had sent me my favorite pie....her internationally renowned and known Coconut Cream pie....It is yummy on yummy. Thanks Beverly. I can't believe you sent the whole pie. Usually she keeps half the pie for Jimmie

Got a package from Mayon and Mackie Weeks of inspirational books, a book Mayon wrote of the songs he had written and some CD's, what classy people. (Thanks Mayon and Mackie). Mayon's inspirational card was....on the front it was a doctor saying "We will be treating your cancer with chemo, radiation and whoop-ass, open the card and it says..."Whatever to WHOOP it into remission'" I've been working with Mayon on his acting and I believe he's coming along fine...don't ya'll.

John and Peggy Hood also sent a care package. It

consisted of some DVD's and a bottle of very expensive wine. The package that the wine came in even said...Very Expensive Wine! Both John and Peggy have been very supportive with several issues I've had to deal with over the last year. Thanks John and Peggy.

Gary and Brenda brought some prescriptions that I needed to be filled; I guess I'll have to pay for that. Not anything important, just some eye drops that Dr. Barbara Ciampa told me I would have to use the rest of my life. I asked her what would happen if I didn't use them and her response was. Let's see....you're already blind in one eye and if you don't take the drops, you will have twin eyes....blind in both. I think I will continue to use them! Dr. Ciampa also told me I had a Cadillac....I told her I did not, I had a Lexus.

Got cards from Cheryl & Hector Ray (Mr. Eagle), John & Peggy, and a beautiful note from my Daughter & grandson....Caden. What a cutie that boy is!
 And what a wonderful 1st birthday party we had.

Many others have not sent a care package yet, so use this as a reminder. Because of your tardiness, I will expect each package to be at least $50 in value. I will be checking the prices. Just check with Brenda, she knows the next person coming down here from Fayetteville. I will also check with Brenda to see who's asking her!!!

Several people have questioned my spelling. Well, they are only typo's, and no, my spell check does not work on this document for some reason. I am really a pretty good average spelllerrrrr.

Wow, what a long day with the early appointment, golf and a late dinner.

Good night everyone.

<u>June 30, 2012 (Saturday)</u> **Peaches, Tomatoes and Handcuffs**

After a few coffees we went out to breakfast. After breakfast, we headed to historical downtown Fernandina Beach. What a beautiful area and they were having a farmers market right in the middle of town. We purchased peaches and fresh tomatoes. Everything went well except for one small situation. I was arrested for solicitation. After they looked at my driver's license and saw my age, they took the handcuffs off. I told them I was just looking for a dinner date so Gary, Brenda and I would have a fourth. Drove back to Amelia Island for lunch, then back home. I looked at my watch and said "hey, its nap time, we were all tired from eating. Well maybe just a little of Beverly's coconut pie!!

The nap was great, then a walk on the beach. That was calm as I've ever seen the ocean. I'm guessing it was because of the heat and almost no wind at all. After finishing our walk on the beach went to the pool for a bit (so we would not have to take a bath later) and then got home and called a restaurant for reservations. We had to leave a message, but asked for an 8 pm reservation. When they called back, they said they were very busy, would we mind coming at 8:30....I said, no, not at all, if you don't mind us coming in our pj's. The restaurant is called Joe's 2nd street Bistro in downtown Fernandina beach. All of us are looking forward to the dinner. Kind of like Yogi Berra said, people don't go there anymore, because you can never get a seat.

 Finally 8:30 we arrived and were seated. The dinner was outstanding. If I keep this up, I will not be able to fit into the body mold I have to get into each day for my treatments. Oh well, I guess they can make another…

Good night everyone.

Chapter 13

A Journey With Me

Week 3

<u>July 1, 2012 (Sunday)</u> **Golf Hall of Fame**

Kind of a lazy day. Gary and I went to the golf course and hit some balls but it was extremely hot. Not as hot as I hear it is in Fayetteville, but hot on hot. Got back and decided to cook breakfast and have some of the fresh tomatoes we purchased yesterday....just the usual, eggs, bacon, grits, toast and a side order of pecan waffles with plenty of butter, just a little something to get the cholesterol up a little.

Headed to St Augustine, to the Golf Hall of Fame. This place is something else, and to me, the most impressive part is the trophies of the four majors at the top of the tower. Kind of tickled to see Raymond in there since he is from Fayetteville. Also a lot on Bob Hope which I enjoyed also.

After the Hall of Fame, we drove to a very historical downtown St. Augustine, Fla. Oldest city. At this time it was so hot we didn't do a lot of outside sight seeing and then drove back to Amelia Island to get ready for dinner.

Going to Baxter's tonight. At dinner Brenda, Gary and I met another couple that lives here in Amelia Island.

Bernie and Joy, nice couple and as it turns out, they are very good friends with Ethan, my friend that is getting us on Long Point Golf Course tomorrow. We are both really looking forward to that, it is a premier course here and two of the holes run along the ocean.

Joy is having a tough go with breast cancer and taking the same Chemo I took almost 17 years ago. She had a great attitude and was a very pleasant lady.

Later on, another couple came in and Joy introduced us to them. Another nice couple and the husband was 91 years old. I couldn't believe it, he was in remarkable shape. He also said he was buying anyone a drink that was 90 or older.....there were no takers. Had a great dinner that included those green fried tomatoes with shrimp, OUTSTANDING!

Tomorrow is coming early, my appointment treatment is at 7:15, which means I will have to drink my 32 oz.'s of water at 6:30. This also means I will have to get up sometime around 5 am.

Good night everyone.

July 2, 2012 (Monday) **Brotherly Love and Golf School**

You talk about bad news, good news. Bad news...I was in Jacksonville before 6am.....Good news....I was all done with my treatment by 7:30am and had the whole day to do whatever I wanted.

Made a new friend today, her name was Terry, her husband was in for his treatment and she and I had a wonderful conversation. She was talking about the First Baptist Church in Jacksonville. She said they had 211 members in the choir...wow. What a wonderful person and she put everything in perceptive. Frankly, she picked me up; her husband was a Chaplin in Atlanta at the prison. Her outlook on life was just wonderful. I enjoyed her conversation very much.

Gary and I had a tee time at 10:30 at one of the finest golf courses I have ever played. It's called Long Point at the Plantation. Absolutely beautiful and in great shape. Two of the holes ran right along the Atlantic Ocean...what scenery all over the course. The fairways were like hitting it off carpet, and the greens were smooth and fast. I'm not going to tell you what I shot...yes I will, I shot 78 and Uncle Gary came in second. Gary said I'm not here for treatments, but rather attending a golf school. What a sore loser he is.

Baxter's for dinner....love that place. Met the owner Michael tonight and what a pleasure he was. I told him how much his restaurant made me feel at home. Very friendly employees and a great clientele. Just friendly people that have made me feel even more comfortable.

Tonight I had shrimp, scallops, and grouper....yummy. Can't wait for Gary and Brenda to leave so I can get back to my normal dinners....salad. After all, I still need to fit that body cast for my treatments. Obviously kidding, their visit has made my purpose here more at home. And best of all, Gary came in second...did I say I kicked his butt on the golf course?

Appointment in the morning at 7:30.

Good night everyone.

July 3, 2012 (Tuesday) **Tightey Whities**

Early morning, off to Jacksonville for my 7:30 appointment. Chatted a little with the lady (Terry) I met the other day while drinking my water. (32 oz.'s if I haven't mentioned that earlier) She introduced me to her husband Joe. Joe asked me how my wife was dealing with this....I lost it for a bit. They called Joe back and then came to get me. Good morning BOB.

Literally a day of rest. Gary and I went to hit some golf balls at the golf course then went home and got Brenda to go and do some shopping. Our goal was to go to the most expensive shops in the area and spend, spend, and spend. Trust me; there are some really expensive stores here.

Our first stop was at TJ Max....Brenda went in there saying she was going to buy the most expensive slacks they have....so she did. We then drove to the king of expense....Wal-Mart. Gary only brought one pair of underwear with him, so he figured he needed to have some clean ones on to drive home in the morning....bought a package of three. Tightey Whities....you got to be kidding me. Finally Gary went overboard; he purchased a white Rolex watch. When he gets home, ask him if he is wearing Brenda's watch.....looks like it!

Had lunch at a place called Parkville Grill....we all had Ruben sandwiches? Maybe the best Ruben I've ever had....did I mention the French fries? Have you ever noticed how a Ruben sandwich makes you sleepy...I have? Oh well, nap time here on Amelia Island.

One of the nice things about having a sister in law that is in the hair business, yes she does hair, and yes she did mine.

Just a little trim and cleanup of the neck hair. I hope it last me for the duration of my treatments, but I don't think it will....maybe I'll grow a pony tail while I'm here. Yes, that's it, a pony tail and some sort of small ear ring.

Then all I'll have to do is learn how to play a guitar and sing.

Big dinner tonight. Hot dogs, chips or potato salad. That is definitely within my income level. Does potato have a toe on it; I don't believe so, potato. If it did have a toe on it, would you have to keep it trimmed?

Sure do miss my Mello Mango!!

I got an email from our fine Pastor, John Cook and he said after reading my Journal that it proved I was certified....what does that mean? I know I'm not a Certified Public Accountant or anything like that, but it sure makes me feel important.

Good night everyone.

July 4, 2012 (Wednesday) **His Footprints**

Contrary to popular belief, I do have a serious side to me and it surfaced this morning. The next few days will be very tough. Today is the anniversary of the day Scottie got sick and tomorrow is the day she passed. She taught me so much for which I will always be thankful. She would have loved being with me here, I can see her right now, curled up in a chair with one of her favorite authors reading away, and she loved the ocean so much.

I know God has his plan, and I don't question it, but I miss her so much. I honestly feel like I have lost a big part of my heart, and it aches. I am thankful to God for the 44 plus years that we had together. Thanks so much for those of you that are praying for me, I'm a living example of the fact that prayer does work...what an AWESOME GOD we have. I can't even think of all the ways He has blessed me, but I'm grateful to have had Him by my side all the way, and I know he is now. As the poem says, those are His footprints in the sand as he carries me and my family through this and I take great comfort knowing that.

Gary and Brenda were delightful and a sight for sore eyes. They have just left for Fayetteville and I wanted so much to be following them home. I sure do miss my home.

Went to get the car cleaned up and the grocery store. I was going to eat leftovers for lunch but stopped by the local deli and had a great chicken sandwich, they had someone there cooking it on the grill for the 4th. When I pulled back into the plantation, they were having a parade. Everyone had their golf carts decorated for the 4th.

Of course, chicken makes me sleepy so took a great nap. When I got up I decided to take a walk on the beach. It was so nice, lots of people there(very nice scenery). A nice breeze was blowing, making it very comfortable being outside. I know it's been hot in Fayetteville, but in the high 90's here. The breeze on the beach does make it cooler I might add.

Baxter's for dinner......**Good night everyone.**

July 5, 2012 (Thursday) **Dr. Wilson, It Is**
Early treatment today...7am and then my weekly appointment with the doctor. He basically says, how you doing, any problems or concerns, how's your golf game and that's about it. I would really like to know how much he gets paid for that 5 to 7 minute talk.

Gary called and said he had left his hair dryer here. He did remember to pack his make-up, but left the dryer. You folks in Fayetteville may not see him out anywhere soon because of that. He never leaves home without doing hair and make-up! Maybe he will look more like me now.

Someone said to me one day, Jerry, why don't you ever comb the back of your head, my response was, because I can't see it. I sure hope Bill Kirby doesn't read this paragraph.

Read a sermon my former pastor sent me on grief this morning. It sure shed some light for me on this subject. It also mentioned that our Lord grieved also, as weird as it may sound, it's comforting to just know that. I guess we all will at one time or another. My current pastor and friend John Cook also called this morning and assured me that God was taking care of Scottie...I can't think of a better care taker. (Keith and Kimberly just like the dragonfly story!)

Several years ago I was having lunch at Highland Country Club by myself and the waitress came up and said what I can get for you Dr. Gilbert (Dave Gilbert). Well of course I'm not Dave but he and I have joked about it over the years.

Today while I was hitting golf balls, one of the owners came up to me on the driving range and said, Dr. Gates, before you leave would you stop by the pro shop so we can discuss your billings. I told her I was not Dr. Gates, but I did play a Dr. one time on TV. Dave Gilbert played a major influence on me taking this type of treatment because of a paper he wrote on Prostate Cancer and Proton Treatments.

Had a great lunch...Asian salad with shrimp. Water to drink...you would think I'm tired of water having to drink 32 oz. before each treatment. Do Asian salads make you sleepy? They do me, looks like nap time.

Nice nap, now off to the beach for a walk. Plenty of people still on the beach (more scenery) must be vacationers for the July 4th week. Great breeze, making the walk very pleasant. Met one guy fishing, he was fishing for whiting and anything he could catch. I'm going to have to go to Wal-Mart this weekend to get a rod and some hooks. Looking forward to seeing all the interesting people there.

Having dinner in tonight I thought, it's been a rough two days. My blood pressure was even extremely high when I saw the doctor today, but we got through it. Did you see those footprints in the sand....they were not mine.

Good night everyone.

<u>July 6, 2012 (Friday)</u> **Towel Washing**

Met a fellow yesterday from Charlotte, N.C. and his wife. They were going back to Charlotte for the weekend but had a 9:20 treatment time. I suggested they trade with me (7:20) and they could get an early start on their trip.

They did and I believe I'm going to change my preferred time. I'm getting tired of getting up at dark thirty.

Treatment went well today and BOB told me to have a good weekend. By-the-way, blood pressure went back to normal 124/76, felt much better about that. It was so high Thursday that I can't even count that high!

Time to do a little cleaning; I am somewhat anal in that area as some might know, but as my mother used to say, cleanness is next to Godliness and that's good enough for me. Washed sheets, pillow cases, towels and a few golf shirts. How often are you supposed to wash towels and sheets?

I have a friend in Fayetteville, (she knows who she is) that washes her towel every time she uses it. Is that normal or nuts. I think its nuts. Hey, I have an idea. When someone tells me how often I'm to change sheets, I'll just turn them around since I only sleep on one side....works for me.

Off to the driving range to work on my game, and it needs it. However, I did manage to beat Gary when he and Brenda were here. That will carry me for a while.

Had a wonderful nap. I'll never know how I was able to get along without that daily rest and work at the same time.

Rested now and off to the beach for a grinding, grueling, gut wrenching walk. Walked for a total of 55 minutes, no telling how far I walked, it must have been at least two miles....wonder if that is a record. I did walk at a faster than usual pace which is good, but occasionally had to slow down to admire the scenery...you know, the ocean, sand dunes, buildings etc.

Ok folks, some of you are falling down on the job. Living here in war like conditions I was expecting more care packages.

(Everyone knows I'm kidding here I hope)...Got home from my grueling walk and did have a care package from Susan. And I mean a care package...listen to this. Rosemary and Currant Biscotti. Dried Cherry and Almond Granola. Roasted pecans and Cheese Biscuits, and a Sour Cream Pound Cake...now that's a care package. I don't know what any of it is (And all of you must be impressed with my spelling of each item, don't be, Susan labeled everything and even told me what to have it with) Susan thank you so much. As most of you know she has been a shining light in the Lighthouse

Sunday School Class, and does so much to help others. Oh, and I love the new CD by Giles, it's beautiful.

How do you thank everyone? I've stretched my brain for a way I can repay everyone for all the wonderful thoughts, phone calls, emails and prayers. There is no doubt God knew what he was doing when he got me back to Fayetteville and Snyder Memorial Baptist Church. From every fiber of my heart and soul.... I thank you!!!! But yet that just doesn't seem like enough.

OK, out to Baxter's for dinner, I just love that place and the food is outstanding. Met a young couple (early 50's I'm guessing) and had an absolute ball. Gary and Judy were their names, and for some reason, the three of us just hit it off with each other and had a lot of laughs. You know, laughing is the best medicine in the world and doesn't cost a dime. Speaking of laughter, Becky sent me a clip of Andy Griffith, "What it is, Is Football". I remember the first time I heard that for some reason. Gary and I were at our cousins (Albert, Cecil) house and I remember laughing until crying. Then we went outside and played tag. What wonderful memories. I also heard a preacher was doing a sermon on "What I Learned by watching the Andy Griffith Show". Do you think we could talk John Cook into doing that?

Whoa, it's almost 10pm,

Good night everyone.

July 7, 2012 (Saturday) **Al Capone's Hit Men**

Up at 6am, not because I wanted to, just woke up and was wide awake. I almost called a few of you folks but decided that could be upsetting to some of you.

Messed around here a little, a little TV and some time on

my laptop and then went to hit some golf balls to kill the morning. After lunch went for a walk on the beach, I'm still guessing about two miles. That's four days in a row and I'm beginning to feel the effects.....good feeling, sure hope I keep it up. It's now about 2pm and thinking about going for a swim in the pool....but don't want to overdo it all in one day. OK, thought about it and a nap won out. Nap time folks.

Out to dinner, back to Baxter's for their steak sandwich, one of the best I've ever had. But most important, I've never spent a dull moment there. Always have met someone interesting and tonight was no different.

Met this woman from Chicago. She comes to the Island ten days each month of the year. Her husband is a lawyer in Chicago. Wonder if he knows Al Capone. She told me she was a jock and enjoyed all sports, but was particularly interested in golf. I told her I was an athletic supporter myself. OK, everyone knows where this is going. Yes I'm hitting balls with her in the morning and playing 9 holes on one of my favorite golf courses, Long Point.

Long Point is absolutely beautiful, and as I've mentioned earlier in this journal, two of the holes run along the Atlantic Ocean.

If I get shot on the golf course by one of Al Capone's hit men, it has been nice knowing everyone, and I sure will miss you. On second thought, I believe I'm going to carry my Smith and Wesson 38 with me. All of you know that I was Barney's assistant.

Good night everyone.

Chapter 14

A Journey With Me

Week 4

<u>July 8, 2012 (Sunday)</u> **Peanut Butter, mayo, Banana's and Aunt Marjorie**

My friend from Baxter's...Wendy called and asked if I wanted to meet her at Long Point and hit some balls and maybe play if it didn't get too hot. Well folks, enjoyed the driving range...well equipped and laid out well. First class you might say...hit irons, and driver, chipped a bit and putted some. I told her I would give her a chance by putting left handed....I always putt left handed. Way too hot to play so she showed me some secrets of how to better get around on the Island...they were very helpful.

Practiced for about an hour and a half and then went home to one of my favorite sandwiches in the world. Chunky peanut butter, mayo and bananas....add some chips and tea and that's what I call a wonderful meal.

My aunt Marjorie could slice a banana better than anyone I've ever seen....they just don't make talent like that anymore. Oh, just for the record, if my new friend here, Wendy, played my neighbor and dear friend Helen...my money would be on Helen. After all, Helen is one of the best putters I've ever seen. Not to mention my other friend is 91!

I don't know if banana sandwiches make you sleepy, but they sure do me...nap time.

After nap spent about ten to fifteen minutes by the pool and had to get in twice....hot on hot here. I know it is in Fayetteville also. It's so hot here I had to have a piece of the Sour Cream Pound cake Susan sent me. Put a few strawberries on it....awesome. Thanks again Susan. I believe it brought down my body temperature a bit....you think?

Dinner time, not sure what I will do tonight. I've got to get up at dark thirty in the morning to be at my appointment with BOB at 7am. Tomorrow my son is flying down to work in this area and I will be able to spend a little time with him. He will be working in Jacksonville and on down to Orlando during the week.

Just as a note of interest, a friend, Mr. Kirby emailed me and asked if I had a blog. My response was, no, I think I have prostate cancer, but the doctors have not mentioned a blog. I'm going to ask the doctors about that blog thing in the morning. I went on to say, I don't even know how to spell blog. Mr. Kirby has incorporated this journal on his blog for those of you that know what that is. Enough said about this. Of course Mr. Kirby is with the paper and arguably a great putter. Thanks Bill (you have been a friend for many, many years) for your interest, it's much appreciated. I also will never forget the respect and kind words you used to write about Scottie, she was your friend also.

Another wonderful night at Baxter's, the food was outstanding and the company even better. My friend Windy was there and she introduced me to her friend Patt, yes with two t's, that's not a misspelling!..I love these people; they talk about helicopters, helicopter pads and the repairs they are having to make to theirs at their homes. They talk about the south of France and Morocco.....finally I said, has anyone ever been to Apex or Holly Springs.....ha, ha....no one had! All kidding aside, these are such friendly people and I've really become attached to them all. They have welcomed me into their fold....especially when they found out I was the Prince of Wales, once removed.

Its late, **good night everyone**, really miss you all!

<u>July 9, 2012 (Monday)</u> **Father and Son**

Well, got up at 5 this morning for my 7am appointment. When I got there and continued drinking my water, they came out and said the gantry was down and they were running about 45 minutes behind.

Then they said, Mr. Wilson, do you think you can hold it that long. My response was, can you leap tall buildings and stop a train...no I can't hold it. Drank more water to keep me up to par and was getting a little angry at the delay. Then these two couples came in with their children. I introduced myself and found out they were from England.

One from London and the other from Newcastle. One child was 15 months, the other was 23 months and they were there for some type of cancer treatment. (I never ask unless they discuss it as to what type) Two small children with cancer, it broke my heart and I slapped myself all the way home just for getting a little angry.

 The first time I ever met Scottie, she had a saying on her mirror, and it said....I used to complain because I had no shoes, until I saw a man that had no feet. I deserved being slapped, and should have been slapped hard.

Isn't it funny, the last sentence in my devotional this

morning was, 'Sit quietly in My Presence, letting my thoughts reprogram your thinking?' God has to reprogram me often!

Young Mr. Wilson flew in today for a visit and combination working in the area, even going to Orlando to see some customers in that area and work with a few of their sales reps. He and I walked out on the beach and took my two mile walk....not bad, twice in one day. Where are they holding those Olympic trials anyway? I might want to try out for the two mile beach walk.

About time for Dinner and I think I will take Keith to Baxter's....worried however, my reputation there is not very good....so what… going anyway.
We had a wonderful dinner at Baxter's. I introduced Keith to everyone that I've met, including the owner...Michael....but it's pronounced Michelle. Glad he's call Michelle instead of me. We had a great dinner, and had a wonderful evening. A lot of good laughs and he even saw Miss Gold Olympic winner from Canada. She was dressed in a full length Pink dress and her husband had white pants and a pink shirt. Some of you will not like that, but they are very classy people.

They also got to meet a very classy young man, my son.

Good night everyone, early appointment....7 am again.

<u>July 10, 2012 (Tuesday)</u> **Witness Protection Plan**

It's now 8:30 am and I'm back from my treatment and ready for the day. Keith and I had a great dinner last night and he got to meet a few of my out of town friends at Baxter's. We had a wonderful time.

There is a lady that comes in with her husband each morning (for treatments) and plays the piano (A Baby

Grand in the lobby waiting area). The other day I asked her if she could play Rachel's Song which is my all-time piano piece favorite. She was not familiar with it. This morning she had the sheet music for it and played it for me. How nice and thoughtful is that, what a classy lady. She plays the piano and organ for her church and a very talented person. She also likes to work with the children that are here for treatment and teach them a little about music. She introduced me to a new song for me called "You Are Mine" by David Haas. She told me to look it up on U-tube and I did. What a beautiful song and David Haas has a great voice. Take a minute and look it up, you will enjoy it very much or I will give you your money back.

Keith will be gone until Thursday night working in the Orlando area, so today I'm going to play golf with a few friends from Baxter's, one of the nicer courses on the Island, It's simply called....The Club.

On the way over for treatment I pass over several bridges. Two of the bridges are very long and overlook the Amelia River and the great Atlantic Ocean. This morning on the way back the sun was shining brightly over the River and Ocean....what a view...How could anyone not know that there is a most creative God? One of the bridges is a draw bridge....I catch myself saying, I sure hope they closed it all the way!

Hey folks, I keep telling you, I'm not a bad speller, just a bad typist. What you are seeing is strictly typos. One person in particular (I will not mention her name) was given the name Anna, so that even if she spelled it backwards, it would still be correct. TYPE-O'S

Matt from Baxter's set up the golf at The Club and it was nice on nice. At least equal to Long Point where Gary and I played. It's located on the Ritz Property. Two other fellows joined us from Baxter's also, Bobby and Chris. As much as I enjoyed the golf, it was some kind of hot...I bet I lost five pounds in water but drank a lot of water and Gatorade. Shot 81 which is not too bad being on a completely new course.

Off to dinner at Baxter's....I keep waiting for them to call me NORM, like on cheers every time I go in. This particular night I got the scare of my life. I was sitting there minding my own business and eating a fish sandwich. The lady from Chicago came in and asked if she could join me.

She is the one with the big attorney husband in Chicago. We start talking and Mike (who works there) comes over and says, Jerry your last name is Wilson, right. I said, it is, and he said I had a phone call on the land line...not my cell phone. My first thought was oh no, something is terribly wrong for someone to call me here on a land line. I said hello and this strange voice, trying to act like they were one of Al Capone's hit men said (I was so nervous about what the call could be about that this may not be exactly what happened, but its close) Hey, I don't appreciate you hanging around with my wife! What, are you talking about, I haven't messed around with anyone, and especially your wife, we just hit golf balls one day.

Well, it was Jay, Stafford, Diane and David pulling one over on me. Yes, they got me good, very good, but don't let them know that. I believe I'm going to see the local sheriff and see if I can get into some kind of "Witness protection Plan" for the rest of my stay here.

Four incredible and wonderful people that I think the world of......and David, I'm not going to mention the fact that Diane keeps calling me, please tell her to stop, it's becoming annoying. Oh, and Stafford, you left your toothbrush over at the house, you want me to just throw it out!! My heart swells just with the thought of you four, I love you all.

I had said earlier that I was now the Prince of Wales....well I misspelled Wales....its Whales.

One last thought before its time for me to go to bed. When the Ocean is at low tide....where does all that water go?

Good night everyone.

<u>July 11, 2012 (Wednesday)</u> **"What is Paranaque?"**

Today is going to be a quiet day, just going to relax all day. Playing golf in 105 index heat wore me out. Maybe some of it is the treatment, but most I suspect was from that heat yesterday. Today, no golf, no walking, just relaxing and resting for my game of Paranaque, which I'm playing tonight at 5:30 just a few miles away at Fernandina Beach.

Yes, that's right, a game of Paranaque with my Life styles of the rich and famous friends who invited me to join them.

By the way, the writer John Grisham is building a home down here. He's even adding a little guest house next door right on the Oceans front, maybe he will invite me to stay there sometime....not.

My first response was, what is Paranaque? They said it's the French version of Bocce...now I completely understood...what is Bocce? Why they invited me, I don't know. They probably recognized some athletic ability (not like Wayne and Hooper) not a lot, but just a little.

OK, here is how it's played. You are on a dirt field of about 25 x 25. There are 3 or 4 players on each team. You stand in a little circle and throw out a little round ball made of some type of cork....it's called the pig. Then you take turns throwing these balls about the size of a baseball, but made of metal and somewhat heavier. You try to get close to the pig. Our team made a comeback and won the game 13 to 10. Afterwards we all went to dinner on the dock overlooking the Amelia River...what a view, the dinner was excellent also. The huge sailboats and motor boats were unbelievable. I often wonder....how someone has a real home somewhere else, a summer mansion here and a boat that probably cost over a million dollars. The only thing I could come up with is....they probably earned it the old fashion way, they inherited it, were drug dealers or somehow related to Bob Bryan my uncle. Regardless, I had a nice time and nice dinner. Time for bed.

Good night everyone.

<u>July 12, 2012 (Thursday)</u> **Frank Upchurch, an Inspiration**

Today it's a 7 am appointment and BOB was not in a good mood. I don't know if he had had a bad night or what. I do know this; he is no longer at the top of my friend list. He is going to have to change his attitude a little.

Met young Mr. Easton this morning. He is 23 months old and was with his mom and Nana (grandmother). They were very nice and from Marietta Ga., where we lived for 14 years. Easton has a brain tumor and has had surgery to remove it. The Proton treatments are to help prevent it from coming back as it is likely to do, let's pray it doesn't. He has to be put to sleep for each treatment so there is no movement at all. The Proton Treatment was recommended because it does not exit damage. It simply

115

goes to the tumor and stays there, preventing, in Easton's case, no further damage to the brain. I ask each of you to put young Mr. Easton on your prayer list. He is a real cutie.

Got a call from Gary this morning and he said he has checked with his Mafia friends in Chicago....I'm safe, I'm on no one's hit list...wheeew! However, David...Diane continues to call....help me please.

Failed to mention my singing debut this morning. Nancy, a woman that comes in with her husband who has his treatment two ahead of me plays the Baby Grand and sings a little. I went over and sat with her and sang a little. (No Mayon Weeks for sure) There were only three or four patients there, not the crowd I wanted. When her husband came out her comment was, Jerry made a joyful noise this morning. The more I thought about that, I was afraid the key word was noise!

Met with the Dr. after my treatment and again he said, any problems, I responded no, any questions; I responded no, ok, I'll see you next week. I swear, I believe I could do his job and maybe even better.

Stopped by Amelia River on the way home to hit some golf balls. It was a beautiful day with a very nice breeze blowing and very pleasant to hit a bag of balls. Saw and spoke to John, one of the guys I played that new game of oops, forgot what it called, anyway, nice guy.

After getting home put on my walking shoes and headed for the beach. It was gorgeous, blue skies, nice breeze and very few people on the beach. Just for future knowledge of my walking...I do jog for about 50 yards of the three miles I'm up to now. At record pace I might add, just to get the ticker running a little faster. Got back to the house and decided to go to the pool for a bit. I'm

working on my Olympic stroke to hopefully qualify next year. You may be familiar with it....it called the dog paddle! Woof, woof it's improving. Keith will be back tonight from Orlando, will probably take him to the restaurant on the dock, can't think of the name of it. Maybe the Waterway Cafe? Not sure.
Did a little cleaning...you know the basics? Not going to tell you what Charlotte Griffin calls me relative to my house cleaning. It's not very nice. I'm not bad at it at all.

My day was made today with a call from Frank Upchurch, what a guy. He has been such an inspiration to so many and is really fighting a battle. I admire him so much!

For those of you that don't know him, please add him to your prayer list....and pray until you sweat! Great guy.

He is taking his treatments in Atlanta, not the same kind of cancer as mine, and quite frankly, I have it easy. He's dealing with that nasty chemo. Been there, done that, and even got a t-shirt and hat.

Keith finally showed up, he had been in Orlando and Sarasota, so he came in from a 5 hour drive. Went to dinner on the Dock called Brett's Waterway cafe. It was awesome, and the view was very nice.

We got to talking about Andy Griffith and I ask him if he had ever heard the tape "What it is, is Football". Becky sent me an email with it and we laughed out loud listening to it this evening. What a great entertainer. He will be missed dearly.

I don't really want to get started with something like this, but could not help it. Keith shared this with me tonight and I thought it was worthy of passing along. Do you know the last thing a Redneck says before he

Dies.............."Hey ya'll, watch this)!!!!!!!! Sorry folks.

Really late now, almost 10 pm. My treatment in the morning is 7:25

Good night everyone.

<u>July 13, 2012 (Friday)</u> **"You Are Mine"**

Oh No, it Friday the 13th.....you know what that means. It's my 19th treatment and we are half way home. Only 4 more weeks left. So Friday 13th is a lucky day as far as I'm concerned.

Keith is riding over to the treatment center with me this morning and I'm going to introduce him to BOB! Sure hope he's in a better mood than yesterday....he probably will be, its Friday, and if you think about what his job consist of.....he gets the weekend off also.

Did not know they would let Keith in the treatment room, but they did. He even took some pictures which I will share with you later on today hopefully. BOB was much friendlier today; he was probably just showing off for Keith. Things went very well today.

Nancy, the lady that plays the piano each morning and is here with her husband (He was having treatment also) let me join in with her again this morning and we sang..."You are Mine". Be sure and look it up on U-Tube, by David Haas....it's a beautiful, beautiful song. By-the-way, she told Keith that I had the voice of an angel.....His comment was that she had to be on some type of Medication....don't know for sure???
Concerning my question as to where the water goes in the ocean when it's low tide, I've only gotten a few responses. It seems the best one is, they pull the plug on the other side....from Susan. Makes perfectly good sense

to me.

My friend from Floyds Knobb, Indiana flew in today to spend a few days with me and I'm looking forward to taking he and Keith to Baxter's tonight. Frank and I were neighbors in Atlanta years ago and we usually get together twice a year. We would go out there once and they would come to see us once a year. One year Frank and I almost won the Highland Member Guest. They don't come any better than Frank and Carol. Carol was Scotties best friend. First class people, just ask Beverly.

Don't believe this, but was disappointed at Baxter's tonight. It was standing room only and we had to sit in a booth...too crowed for me, but dinner was outstanding.

Keith goes home in the morning. We really had a great time, a lot of laughs and fun. He also learned a new breathing technique for golf and where they are building the new Wal-Mart in Fayetteville. It was great he got to go with me to the treatment....I really enjoyed his company and friendship. Sure glad he takes after his mother.

Up late tonight, almost 9:30.

Good night everyone.

July 14, 2012 (Saturday) **Frank, Banana Sandwiches and Elvis**

Said goodbye to Keith and of course walked with him to the car, what a great kid....Love him and Kimberly both.

Frank and I went to the Grill and had breakfast and then went to hit some golf balls. He wanted some help with his swing. After watching him for about a half hour...I said, Frank, I believe I would lay off for about two weeks and then give the game up. He and I are going to play Amelia River tomorrow at 2:30....weather permitting.

Got home and went for a walk on the beach. Must have done 3 plus miles today and it felt good. Frank got some sand in his shoes and took them off to wash them out in the ocean. You know what's funny.....watching a 65 year old man try to put his shoes on standing up with nothing to hold on to. Finally after laughing, I went over and gave him a shoulder to hold on to. Always something funny going on in this life I believe.

Lunch time and I asked Frank if he had ever had a banana sandwich, he said no...Never had Elvis Presley's favorite sandwich in his life. I made a couple sandwiches and we had lunch. He said it was not one of his favorites, but later on he started singing like Elvis.

Drove over to Fernandina Beach to have dinner at Brett's on the River. Frank had the Shrimp Alfredo and I had the Crab Cakes. We then went on the boardwalk to pick out a boat. Pictures will follow.

Stopped by Baxter's to see if Chris was there and wanted to play golf with us tomorrow. He was, and will.

Just something for you to think about. Here on the Plantation there are two speed limits. One is 15 mph, which I understand. The other is 23mph, this one leaves me clueless.

Good night everyone.

Chapter 15

A Journey With Me

Week 5

<u>July 15, 2012 (Sunday)</u> **What an Awesome God**

Great breakfast, Honey nut Cheerios with fresh
strawberries. It was awesome. Didn't have enough
strawberries for Frank...gave him a banana and he started
singing like Elvis again, but also started bending over,
dropping his arms and puckering up his lips like a
monkey....it was not pretty, and I was about to take him
to the golf course to play with some of my friends from
Baxter's. I was so afraid he would play like a monkey,
but not the case. The weather was beautiful and Frank
played very well. One of the best rounds he has played
in a while...I love to see a golfer play well that I'm
playing with, I get as excited as they do over their
success on the course. Frank shot an 82, now he came in
second, but a great round regardless, and I was thrilled
for him.

Ok folks, I have a problem (Houston, we have a
problem). It has nothing to do with were I'm staying, my
treatment schedule or really anything important....but
folks, where am I going to get my next haircut. Beverly
gave me a haircut before I left Fayetteville on June 17.
Brenda gave me a haircut while she and Gary were here.
Now where? The only place I've seen anyone cutting

hair was at Wal-Mart. Wallllllllmart, are you kidding me.
I may not have any other choice. I will definitely have it
cut 3 weeks before I come home so Beverly can correct it
when I get home. Help Beverly!!! I am so pleased that
there is not a vain bone in my body!!

Ok, eat your heart out. Frank and I are staying home
tonight and cooking in. I am cooking my international
famous spaghetti sauce, which we will have with Angel
Hair pasta.

Frank, cooked something for us to snack on, shrimp
wrapped in bacon. It was yummy on yummy. Dinner
turned out wonderful....the shrimp and the spaghetti
were awesome. Now most of you are probably thinking,
wow, Jerry must weigh 300 pounds by now, but no.
When I checked in for my first treatment, they took all
the vitals and I weighed 176... They take your vitals once
a week; in my case it's on Thursday. Last Thursday, I
weighed in at 174. I believe it's the walking....and
amounts of what I'm eating.

Believe it or not, it is now 7:03pm. I could go to bed right
now, but I believe that's a little too early to go just yet.
My legs were cramping up. The golf and the three plus
mile walk has not been kind to my legs. But I love what
I'm doing. The walking has made me feel so much better
and football practice starts on August 15th, I believe I
want to play this year. (lol, lol) Maybe Wayne will hand
the ball off to me, or at least throw it to me.

Just four more weeks left. I can't wait to get home. This
morning when I was walking I had my Mello Mango
shirt on. Someone ask me what was that and I said a
little store I had opened in Fayetteville serving yogurt. I
said I had this fellow running the business for me by the
name of Jackson. I also thought he was doing a fine job
for me. He and his whole family. Don't you just love

Mello mango.....I do. I can't wait to get back and finish out my free card.

Gary swears I'm here for golf school. I can understand him saying that since I beat his butt good, while he was here. I wish that was the case, but you saw the pictures of the gantry they put me in each day. Doesn't look like a golf school to me. But I thank God each day for his grace and all the wonderful blessings he has given me. This treatment is just one of them. I strongly feel like I have made the right decision and God is driving....not just a passenger. What an awesome God we have.

I got so many emails today talking about what a wonderful sermon John gave this morning about how we must trust in God. Some even said it brought them to tears. Are we blessed with John or what? I think so, and I'm so glad I've worked with him on his delivery....he has really improved with my help....don't you think...I do. God Bless you John, we all love you dearly!!!!

Ok, Louise, everyone is talking about what a wonderful Sunday school teacher you are...I agree. Hey, and it only took a few lessons from me to get you on the right track. God has blessed you so, and I'm in agreement with everyone on how prepared you are with all your lessons. Yes, everyone is also thanking me for helping you also. I must admit, you were very coachable and picked up on it very fast, much faster than John did. I love you and keep up the outstanding work you are doing.

Good night every one...it is so late and I have told enough fibs for today!!

July 16, 2012 (Monday) **Good Things Happen to Good People**

Got my appointments changed to the 9am range and I

believe we will enjoy them a little better....at least, it gives BOB the opportunity for him to wake up and hopefully have his second cup of coffee...blah, blah, blah, blah.....

Frank went with me for my treatment and when we got home, we had a little breakfast, and then went for our 3 plus mile walk....blah, blah, blah, blah.

Folks, the reason I've added the Blah, blah, blah...is because I wanted something more interesting to talk about. After all, I have readers from far and wide that I honestly feel I'm obligated to entertain and amuse, and after all, Bill Kirby has writing cramps and is using my material for you folks.....not.

Somewhat of a boring day, but relaxing and all the usual, breakfast, walk, nap, Baxter's....blah, blah, blah.

OK, folks, sit back and relax...find a comfortable chair and hopefully you will enjoy this story....we did very much. Like the old Andy Griffith show...it also has a story and who knows, you might learn something!

I called my new friend that I've met at Baxter's and she said to me one night, I can get you on any course you want to play, just call me. Well this morning when I called, she was playing bridge and said, could she call me back, sure I said. As we got ready for dinner, I had not heard back from Patt, so I somewhat wrote it off. After all, Frank and I could play Amelia River and it's a very enjoyable, and in good shape course.

We wanted to play Amelia National because of all the nice things we had heard about it. She finally called me back and said Amelia National was off the Island and she had no pull there...so, there you go, no problem at all. See there are two types of people here, Plantation people, and then all the rest. I'm not sure which one I am yet....but working on figuring that out.

Frank and I drive to downtown Fernandina Beach just to walk around and find something that might be interesting for the evening's dinner. Frank was hungry because he missed a banana sandwich for lunch. We stopped at a place called Marina Seafood Restaurant for Frank to get a bowl of oysters. I tasted one and it was good.

Now back to the streets to find something more interesting. We ended up at a place called Irish Gardens. We sat out on the patio, which I thought was beautiful, it even had banana trees scattered around. I bought a nice cigar, which I smoke maybe once a month and we were having a nice conversation and enjoying ourselves. I had to go to the bathroom and when I got back a young lady was sitting at our table...very young, she was three (3). In a few minutes her mom came by with her other daughter and introduced herself as Morgan. She had her other daughter with her and her name was Rieley...a real cutie, in fact, so was mom. Well, McKinnsey, the three year old had taken her shoes off and placed them on the table and really made herself at home. In a few minutes this fine young man shows up and he is the dad.....Joe Parrish. He is also the owner of the place (Not really, McKinnsey is the owner...trust me), and Morgan is his wife along with the two girls Rieley and McKinnsey.

After some conversation, we found out he is a scratch golfer and one of the best on the Island. I ask him if he was familiar with Amelia National, he said yes and the pro there was a friend of his.

He called him, gave us a certificate to play there at a reduced rate to boot. What a great story or at least I think so. McKinnsey finally gave us permission to leave (after all, she was the boss) and we went to the Surf to get a Hamburger and some fried pickles. The entertainment left a lot to be desired, but the hamburger and pickles were awesome. Then we stopped by Baxter's to make sure everyone was ok, then on to home.

This little story also even more confirms the saying which is one of my favorites....<u>Good things happen to good people</u>....I agree. We wanted to play Amelia National and as good people....it happened. All because this little three year old girl took charge.

Good night everyone, and remember......be good!!!!!!

<u>July 17, 2012 (Tuesday)</u> **Nana...What an Inspiration**

Treatment today at 9:30 blah, blah. Oh, by the way BOB and I are not on speaking terms anymore. I don't really know what has got into him, but his attitude is just not what it was.

Everyone remember young Mr. Easton, the 23 month child with the brain tumor. I had the opportunity to speak to his mom and Nana this morning and what wonderful people. They are from the Marietta, Ga. area where we used to live for 14 years. This Nana sat there with a big, big smile on her face and talked about how much she depended on God. What a major role He has played in her life and there was no doubt in her mind, He was going to get Easton through this, and it was going to make them all stronger. What an inspiration just listening to this woman. Never once mentioning herself, and as I left to go back for my treatment, she said they were all praying for me. You know what; I believe young Easton is going to be just fine....don't you? This Nana has lost her husband and mother during the last year. It always amazes me how someone can remain so positive and upbeat while going through such adversarial trials in their life.

A little lunch...blah, blah. Now on the way to Amelia National....what a golf course. I don't know that I have ever played a finer golf course in my life. Everything was just pristine....the fairways, the greens, the sand traps, the scenery, and listen to this....About every 4 or 5 holes they had a box full of iced down water bottles.

Frank and I had a ball; the course was so nice we even forgot how hot it was....well almost. After we played I went into the pro shop and did everything but kiss the pros feet....hoping to get another Invitation....didn't happen. Oh well, what a memory!

Hey, Frank and I saw a pink flamingo tonight on the way home...and he or she was flying....across the bridge. Have you ever seen a pink flamingo flying...we never have? In fact, most of the ping flamingo's I've ever seen was stuck in someone's yard.

At Baxter's tonight my friend was there, Ethan...what a nice guy and he has been very nice to me ever since I've been here.

We had a great conversation and he told me about his time at the University of Pennsylvania. He was quite the athlete. At one time he held several school records on the track team. He was very proud of that fact, and he should be...tonight he said all his records had been broken...by women, we had a great gut laugh over that fact. He didn't have a problem with that at all, but it was a funny moment...he has his head on straight and I think a lot of him. And even more importantly, he's a fine conservative.

While walking today, Frank and I stopped to talk with some people that were playing golf on the Links course here on the Plantation. As it turned out, they (A family) went to school at Wake Forest and were very proud of that fact. They now live in Tenn....I told them I had a friend that pitched the winning game in the College World Series back in 1957; I believe that was the year. I also told them that that same person, Jack McGinley, used to baby sit Gary and me when we were 5 and 6 years old. All kidding aside, I think a great deal of Jack (and enjoy playing golf with him also), and like me, he lost a very beautiful lady (Miss Fayetteville) way too young.

How about this for dinner? Frank and I both had escargot (why does that word have a (t) on the end of it?) and French Onion soup for dinner. Actually I could make a meal just out of the snails...Baxter's does it right.

Got an email today from John saying how much he enjoys reading my journal each day. He said it was somewhat like watching a soap opera..."As the Stomach Turns".

OK, almost 9:30, **Good night everyone**.

<u>July 18, 2012 (Wednesday)</u> **Carol, and Carole, Two of Scottie's Special Friends...and mine!**

Took my friend Frank to the airport this morning on my way to my treatment and we had a wonderful time together. Great conversation, good golf, great food and a lot of laughs. Scottie had two very special friends in her life, Carol Dupont (Frank's wife), and Carole Sallee. (Yes, the second Carole adds an e to her name for all you English majors out there) She was as close to those two people as anyone I've ever seen, and quite frankly, they both are special people to me also. If you looked up the word friends in the dictionary, there would be a picture of all of them together, including Frank. They don't come any better.

Treatment went well....blah, blah. Did meet a new

person this morning. Her name was Lisa and she was there with her mother who has some type of brain tumor. They are from south Florida and her normal doctor started her on chemo. The people at the Proton Center told them the chemo would not work at all on her type of tumor. (Folks, these people here in Jacksonville are doing some wonderful things to young and old alike) Yet, her home doctors, who probably knew that also, started it anyway. It seems to me that someone was waging a life on the line for insurance money...unreal! As I recall, each treatment of chemo I had back in 96 was almost $7,000 a pop.

Good lunch, great nap. Now it's time to go hit some golf balls. Walked outside and it's raining...oops, no practice. I guess its Judge Judy for me, love that woman....she is so funny and tough!

OK, educational time....got an e-mail from Becky today and she used the word...epicurean, anyone know what it means, or better still, anyone know how to spell it? I spelled it right because I copied it from her e-mail. Don't you just love it when these ex-school teachers show off? Just kidding Becky.

Baxter's for dinner. Had dinner with my buddy Ethen and he was telling me about going to see Jersey Boys a few months back in Jacksonville. That has to be an awesome show, I've heard nothing but good things about it. Would love to see the Little Theater in Fayetteville do it. Better still, would love to go to New York to see it....think I will! I had my Masters shirt on and this guy sitting across from me asked me if I had ever been to the Masters (I didn't care for this guy from the get go and didn't like the way he asked me) and my response was, yes, I was even there in 86, the last time Jack won. As we have all done, when I got home I wish my response had been, "Yes, six times, but I only made the cut three of those six"....come on brain start thinking!! Maybe when I get out of golf school here in Amelia Island I will try and qualify.

Hey guess what, I only have 16 more treatments and then I will be home. Please take that as fair warning.

WOW, it's almost 9PM, **Good night everyone**.

<u>July 19, 2012 (Thursday)</u> **Kingsley, Georgia and MacDonald Mustard**

Appointment went well. Saw the Doctor today and I swear, I believe all he said was...."Everything going OK?" Sure Doc. That was pretty much it, another several thousand for him. No Problem....blood pressure was a little high but I blamed it on BOB since I had just had my treatment.

Got an email from Stafford today giving me advice on how to cure the leg cramps that I seem to be having a problem with. She said to steal some mustard packages from McDonald's and put them on the bed stand and eat one as I feel the cramps coming on. Jay, you really need to work with this woman.....steal! OK, Stafford, I got them and did not get caught.

My friend Greg is flying in today to spend a few days. Greg and I go back to little league baseball. He played third base. Of course the real stars back then were the parents. I can see his mother sitting in the stands today.

The boys of 57, what a team (city champs) and what wonderful memories. Gary did a great job of putting together a reunion of that team just a few years back, most of the players were there.

On my way to the airport I stopped at this very

expensive clothing store to see if there was anything I couldn't live without (as Gary would say) and while shopping in TJ-Max the lights went out (bad storm)....where was I when this happened, in the bathroom of course. They asked everyone to come to the front of the store and I hollered out, "I will when I'm done in here." Finally I made it to the front of the store and met some fine people from Kingsley Georgia. The wife said her husband always bought a pair of socks when they went shopping, but she could not figure out why....she said he had a drawer full of socks.

We talked a bit more and I told them I did not care for the city or county they lived in. That's where I got my speeding ticket. She said she was so sorry and was ashamed of their speed trap county. They also said that last year the newspaper wrote that the county made over three million on tickets....they probably don't even have to pay taxes there because of that revenue (hey Tony, now there's an idea for you). She went on to say that they have only lived there for a few years and she had raised their children in Waycross Georgia. I asked her if she knew any Darden's from Waycross. She said oh yes, Mr. Darden started a restaurant called the Green Frog.

Folks, after that, Mr. Darden started a little company called Red Lobster and grew it into the company it is today, later on, sold it to General Mills I believe...not bad huh? Bill Jr. and Cynthia were neighbors of ours for fourteen years in Atlanta. I met Mr. Darden Sr. a few times and what a fine gentleman.

He should have been a senator like me. Cynthia has the most fun, contagious laugh I've ever heard (great medicine). Got to visit with them a few months back when Keith, Luke and I went to the University of Georgia spring game. Had not seen them in eighteen years. Had a ball. Small world huh? By-the-way, this gentleman and wife I was speaking to in the store said he was 87....I've never seen anyone that looked that good at that age....I don't at 67. By-the-way, I purchased a t-shirt for $5.95....overboard I know, but living crazy down here, it must be the treatments!

Anyway, picked Greg up and it was raining cats and dogs here. Because of that we were not able to walk today so we spent the day trying to figure out how we could get Mr. Obama out of office. Greg is very politically astute, as Scottie was and she used to love to have Greg visit us when our class had our reunions...Greg always stayed with us except the one time he stayed with Bill.....Bill he said he enjoyed our home over yours.....Just kidding Bill. I don't believe I mentioned, but Greg now lives in Milwaukee where he is some kind of executive or something like that.
Time for dinner and Greg got to meet all the characters at Baxter's, even Ethan, who is not normally there on Thursday nights. Even the Queen of Ice skating was there with her husband. We both had 6 oz. filets which were wonderful. Red meat is good for you....isn't it?

As you may know or not know, I have a passion for the game of golf. Greg bought me a little book with famous sayings in it that all of you have heard at one time or another. Here's one that I have not heard. "Give me golf clubs, fresh air, and a beautiful partner, and you can keep the golf clubs and fresh air....Jack Benny......I agree!

Oops, after 9pm, on to bed.

Good night everyone.

July 20, 2012 (Friday) **"No Thank you, Jerry"**
Greg went with me for my treatment this morning and I invited him into the gantry so he could see how the treatments are administered....they asked him if he

would like to meet BOB and he politely said, no thank you. I asked Greg what he thought after seeing the gantry, he said, all he could see was the bottom of my feet. Folks, only 15 treatments left.

After Mike got me going on the best route to the treatment center, the view and drive is absolutely beautiful. You pass over about 17 bridges. Got home, and began to get ready to go play golf at the golf school I'm attending. Amelia River is really in good shape and I was looking forward to playing a round of golf with Greg. This was only his 5th time he has played this year and he strikes the ball very well. We had a great time, heat was a bit much, but it got better as a breeze picked up on the back nine. Got home and we both were worn out so no walk today. By-the-way, Greg shot 94 because it was 94 degrees, and the humidity was also 94.

Dinner was going to be my treat and I was going to make baked Ziti for the first time ever. I've had it at Little Italy several times and love it but have never made it before. It was delicious, it could have looked better, but the flavor of my famous sauce was good. Probably should have had a salad with it, but the garlic bread was good also.

Watched a little TV and then bedtime. Greg and I are going to golf school tomorrow and then playing again at Amelia River.

For reasons which I will not go into now, please add Keith's family and the Reif family to your prayer list. Thanks to all of you for doing this.

Anyone who criticizes a golf course is like a person invited to a house for dinner who, on leaving, tells the host that the food was lousy...Gary Player.

Good night everyone.

<u>July 21, 2012 (Saturday)</u> **Hi Ho Silver**

Greg and I went for a walk this morning and it was beautiful, the weather was nice and not too hot. When we got back home, I had a call from my security people and my alarm had gone off at home. Gary went over and everything seemed to be OK. The bad news, Gary got there before the police did. My point here is, why have a monitored home security system, if the Fayetteville police can't get there within fifteen minutes or so. Go figure, the thieves could be in and well gone before the police show up. I'm very disappointed at this moment with the police. Anyone else had this problem in Fayetteville? Hey Tony, help me out here please. I feel like I have been robbed (although Gary said everything was ok), the only thing missing is the horse and mask. Hi Ho Silver.

Don't you just love old people....when Greg and I got back from the golf course I started looking for my cell phone. Could not find it anywhere. Greg said, let's call the course and see if they have it....I insisted there was no way it could be at the course!! After looking and looking, Greg said he was going to dial the golf course and just ask them. How stupid could Greg be, after all I had insisted it was not there. When Mark (course pro) answered the phone at the course he said, oh, Mr. Wilson.....we have your cell phone here....Duh, Duh!!!! Isn't Greg one of the smartest people on this earth....think so.

Stafford, just for your information, the mustard you had me steal from McDonald's has worked. After walking this morning and then going to play golf, my left hamstring was about to cramp. I opened one of my stolen packages of mustard, took it and it worked....thanks. Did you use to be a doctor also?

Drove over to downtown Fernandina Beach for dinner, we went to Brett's on the Waterway. That's where Frank and I bought the two boats. When going over you see some of the most incredible beach front homes you would ever want to see. Driving through historical downtown is very nice also, there are several churches that are beautiful and old on old kind of like my uncle Bob Bryan...I bet he used to attend one of them...you think! Anyway, I had shrimp and Greg had salmon, salmon is not one of my favorite dishes. On the way home stopped at Baxter's to say hello to everyone. Chris and his wife were there, he used to work for the FBI for twenty four years. He also was involved in the President Reagan shooting, but he is one funny guy. He also was the one that took golf lessons and they gave him breathing exercises to use during the swing. Unfortunately, I can't share those techniques here. Trust me, it's funny.

Greg will be leaving tomorrow....I sure have enjoyed his company. We go back a long, long way. We had some great laughs and great conversations. He will be missed. Greg is renting a place for a month in January at Ft. Meyers Florida and invited me to join him for a week....I will be there for sure. How nice it was for him to fly down to spend some time with me.

Understand the Sunday school class is going out to lunch today....sure wish I could be there.

Its late folks, almost 9PM...**Good night everyone**.

Chapter 16

A Journey With Me

Week 6

<u>July 22, 2012 (Sunday)</u> **Cancer is not the End**

Really had a bad night with a horrible dream last night. I
dreamed I swallowed a giant marsh mellow and when I
woke up, I could not find my pillow. Sorry folks, Greg
shared that with me and I thought it was funny.

Just got back from the airport dropping Greg off. We
had a great time but did not like walking back into an
empty house. Oh well, got a crowd coming next week.
Mike, Ray and Gary will be coming down to play some
golf. I know Gary has revenge on his mind. By-the-way,
if he gets lucky and wins, it will not be recorded in this
journal!

One of the conversations Greg and I briefly had was why
this journal, and why I decided to keep track of my
experience here in Florida. Listed below are some of
those reasons, some we discussed, some we did not....

1. To show in some small way the large role Christ
   has played in my life and continues to play.

2. To show others, cancer is not the end...having spent a lot of time with the patients at the Cancer Center in Fayetteville, I've seen a lot of success in beating cancer. Regardless of the type or stage, a good attitude plays such an important role. Having been a stage 4 some 17 years ago is another fact...it can be beaten. Even a little humor doesn't hurt. Does it, Julia, Sue and Pearl, and now Ray
3. Since I can't remember what I had for breakfast this morning, I figured if I didn't write it down, I may not even remember being on Amelia Island.
4. Bill Kirby was having writer's cramps and needed some help with his blog, at least something interesting anyway.
5. Since I have nothing of value to leave my children, this journal, in some way would help them remember me. Just kidding, I do have a Wilson 2000 catcher's mitt, and an old Louisville Slugger 34 inch bat.
6. And lastly, I'm having a ball writing it and getting the responses from everyone. Things like...you have lost it, or, did you fall out of the truck on your head, or, you are completely out of control, and a few others I cannot type here...not really.

This Sunday will be a slow, quiet day, just relaxing today. I will do a little cleaning for the folks coming down this week. Got hungry from the cleaning so went to Harris Teeter and got supplies for making Shrimp Alfredo....it was yummy.

Have a great week everyone....**Good night everyone**.

July 23, 2012 (Monday) **A South Carolina Hall of Famer**

Treatment went well, but I am really getting tired of starting my days off this way....can't wait to get home and get some Mello Mango. That will make everything better.

While driving over today I got a phone call from a very old friend. Ronnie Collins has been a good friend now for over 45 years. We rented a house together before we were married. We had no pictures to hang in this little house on McPhee St.... so we had Bill Kitchens come over and paint a big sun over the couch. That drawing cost us all of our deposit...$50.

Ronnie and I played city basketball for one year, but I really don't remember how the season went. I'm sure with Ronnie being on the team, we must have been good. After all, Ronnie is in the Basketball Hall of Fame at South Carolina. Ronnie is also a member in good standing with the Hall of Shame.

However, I do remember one game in particular where the score was tied with just a few seconds left. We had the ball and called time out. I told the coach to have someone throw the ball to me and I would get it to Ronnie to score. Folks, I had no intentions what so ever of throwing that ball to Ronnie. There was no doubt in my mind who was going to shoot the final and winning shot. Missed!!!! Oh well, we won in overtime. Ronnie and I scored 44 points together, I had 5. I asked Ronnie for his email address so I could send him this journal and he said he didn't have a computer, just call him and tell him what I had written for the day.... That's Ronnie for you!

Great lunch...I had the left over baked Ziti I cooked a few days ago. Then went to the golf course to hit balls, got to get ready for Mike, Ray and Gary. I hope they all bring their pocketbooks. After hitting balls got home and put on my walking shoes). I believe I went past the 4 mile point today. Lookout Stan (my cousin in Roanoke, Va.),

I'm coming after you. Next, maybe the Boston marathon....who knows!!! The sad note today was seeing the American Flag flying at half mask....what a tragedy.

Going to Baxter's tonight for their awesome steak sandwich. Oops, it's almost time for Judge Judy. Someone told me she makes 45 million a year.....? Don't know for sure.

Very small crowd at Baxter's tonight. Had dinner with my friend Ethan. He is going to set up a round of golf for Mike, Ray, Gary and myself at Amelia National for either this Thursday or Friday...what a beautiful course. It's the course that has bottled water for you throughout the course....first class to say the least.

Back home early and probably to bed soon....for whatever reason, it has been a long day. Monday I guess.

Only 14 more and counting. I wonder if Tony will have a ticker tape parade for me upon my return, or maybe Bill Kirby will take me to dinner for doing part of his job for him on his blog.....think not!!! Just a quiet night at home will be wonderful....in my own bed at last.

Good night everyone.

<u>July 24, 2012 (Tuesday)</u> **Mike, Ray, Gary...Let the Games Begin**

Treatment went well...one of the technicians is named Luke (same as my grandson) and I love picking on him. He is an Alabama graduate, and of course I'm a Georgia fan (My son graduated from the University of Georgia)...so we go back and forth with each other. This morning I asked him if he changed BOB into a baseball...he said no, it was an Alabama balloon just saying roll tide. I told him I was going to start pulling for Auburn with Bill Owen. I'll get him back eventually. Great guy he is, and always has a smile on his face.

On the way home decided to get rid of my pony tail and get a haircut. Went into the Wal-Mart but got scared, was afraid I would come out looking like a Wal-Mart shopper you see in those emails. Found a mini-mall with a hair place in it, so stopped there. When I walked in, this Asian lady behind the counter asked if she could help me. I said I needed a haircut and she said she would be serving me this morning....I wanted to say I'm here for a haircut, not a toe or nail job...but I didn't. While cutting my hair she asked if she could trim my eyebrows...I said sure. Then she asked if she could clean up the back of my neck...I said sure. Then I started wondering if this was a a-la-carte haircut, where I had to pay for each item cut. It wasn't, and she did a good job (No Beverly), but a good job none the less. Her business card says her name is Ann Morgan...I wonder what her real name is?

Speaking of Beverly, I called her and ask her, as my hairdresser, to pray for me that I don't come out of this shop looking like Jon or Josh. She said she would, and it helped. Just kidding guys, and thank you both so much for serving this great country of ours. I'm so proud of you both, and I know your Dad and Mom are also.

Talked to Beverly (while asking her to pray for me about the haircut) this morning and she is sending down two Coconut Cream pies with Mike, Ray, and Gary this week. She makes the best I've ever had and I bet none will be left over when these guys leave. Also, Brenda told me to go out and buy some vanilla ice cream because she is sending brownies....so much for this strict diet I've been on. Yep, this fine toned body just might go to the dogs....oh well, what's new.

Dinner at Baxter's, just a salad with baked chicken, but it was good. Had dinner with Eaton, what an interesting man. He has seen and done so many things in his life. Eaton is 77 and I enjoy listening to him talk about all the places he has been and all the important people he personally knows.

Only 13 more treatments before liftoff.

Let the games begin....the boys will be bringing down their golf clubs and we will be playing Amelia National, Long Point and North Hampton.

Late folks, almost 8:30.

Good night everyone.

July 25, 2012 (Wednesday) **Rounding Third and Heading Home**

Treatment went well, then met with the doctor and my two nurses. Vitals were good, blood pressure normal, weight down just a little, 171. (That's for all of you that thought I was eating my way through Amelia Island) I don't believe I've mentioned my two nurses...Tracey and Barbara. They are both very nice and fun and needless to say we cut up a bit. Not bad to look at either. Tracey said she was going to give me a ride on her Harley before I leave and Barbara was telling me they are now treating patients that have gone through the radical surgery when the cancer returns to the area....go figure. Folks, this is good stuff down here and again I'm so glad God directed me to this location and treatment.

I mentioned the boys coming down for golf and let the games begin. Well, just so we are clear on this....it will all be recorded in this journal if I win, lose and no word or documentation at all. And if Gary says he won, don't believe him.

Wandered down to Turtle Cove today. Just another area here on the Island with a nice pool and they serve refreshments. Just walked in like I owned the place and took a lounge chair. Ask the pool girl to please bring me a towel and a chicken salad sandwich, the sandwich was very good...not bad for an old cancer patient. You think they really thought I owned the place? Probably not!

Well, its nap time....got to get up in time to watch Judge Judy and the boys should be here around 6pm...Looking forward to seeing them all.

Boys showed up and I welcomed them to MY summer home here on the Island. I cooked my spaghetti for dinner with a salad and it turned out fine. Can't believe what a picky eater Ray is, I feel sorry for you Joan. Beverly sent coconut pies, Brenda sent brownies and I got another care package from Susan. These guys jumped into Susan's treats and then after dinner, half of one of the pies is already gone. It would not surprise me to see it all gone before morning. We already have had some great laughs and the golf should be fun also. Did you know that Mike used to jump out of airplanes with Frank Upchurch? I asked Frank, why you would jump out of a perfectly good airplane, he said for $55. Each month the army would add it to his $85 monthly paycheck.....boy did they live high on the hog or what?

Tomorrow should be fun, playing my favorite course here, Amelia National. I want Gary to go with me to treatment either Thursday or Friday. I want him to put on the gown and go back to the gantry and see if they will give him the treatment just this one time. We will give it a try and I'll let you know the outcome. I doubt we will be able to pull it off, but if we do, and he gets prostate cancer in the future, he will only have to take 38 treatments vs. 39. You might say, he will have one behind him, just kidding BOB!

A few years back when we lived in Raleigh, I had back surgery. Gary came in and the nurse did not see him come in. He walked out in the hall dressed as he came, and started doing jumping jacks and told the nurse he was ready to go home, he felt fine now....the nurse almost had a heart attack and started to call the doctor, then I walked out in the hall.

Being an old baseball fan, I like what Anna said in her email, I have rounded third and on the way home....sounds good to me, counting tomorrow, only 12 left.

Years ago, the Junior High team went on a bus with the varsity players to Rocky Mount to play them in baseball. Bobby. (Anna's husband) Gary and I all hit home runs that day. It may have been the only home run I ever hit.

OK, it's 9 pm and Uncle Jerry is going to bed.

Good night everyone.

<u>July 26, 2012 (Thursday)</u> **Hi Jerry, You Don't Look so Good Today!**

Special treatment day today. Gary went with me and we did have a little fun at the treatment center. I don't think we look that much alike any more, but several people said, hi Jerry while he was in the waiting room.

They also said, aren't you feeling well today, you don't look so good today....loved it. (Not really) When it was my time in the gantry, Gary walked back with me and put a gown on over his clothes. They all said he could take BOB for me today if he liked, he refused.....wonder why? We all got a big kick out of it, but could not talk Gary into taking my treatment for the day. Hopefully everyone got the picture we took in the Gantry that I sent out earlier.

Folks, I come to you with a very, very heavy heart. Mike and I stood Gary and Ray and we got beat soundly....it was pitiful. But Mike and I tripped getting out of the car as we arrived at the course and twisted our ankles and were greatly handicapped from the get go. We tried our best, but with both of us having swollen ankles it was an uphill battle. Hopefully the swelling will go down by tomorrow....let's hope so!!!!! Of course, it didn't help matters for Gary to shoot a 75 and Ray hitting one in from the sand trap for birdie. Mike and I agreed, you just can't beat black magic....now can you? OK, that's my story and I'm sticking to it!

Tonight dinner at the Ocean Club....that's class on class. Gentlemen wear coats only. Of course Mike is the member and we will be attending as his guest. I sure hope Gary and Ray behave themselves and not embarrass us like they did on the golf course today.

We are home now and the four of us are sitting around in our boxers, not a pretty sight. Gary is ironing his outfit for tomorrow so he will look nice. Dinner was outstanding, really outstanding and we all cut up a little with most of the people there. Met a nice couple from Nashville to start with, a doctor and his wife, they were very nice.

 Now here is the good part.....remember I said, I hope Gary and Ray didn't embarrass us. Ok listen to this....when Gary ordered, he said, I'll have the first thing on the menu, he could not pronounce it so that's how he ordered it. Then later it was Ray's turn. He said, we need to stop on the way home to get some ice cream to put on the coconut cream pie. I'm sorry folks, we can't take either one of these guys anywhere!!! They are so lame! As we left, Mike and I apologized to the staff for our friends and they said, they understood. They said they get people in there like them all the time. However, the two of them were at the top of the list.

Late now folks, almost 9pm.

Good night everyone.

Sending you two pictures, first the picture from our dining room table, and second the winning team....I hope!

<u>July 27, 2012 (Friday)</u> **I Love you Son**

Treatment went well, just ten left....looking forward to getting into single digits. Just realized I haven't said anything about the staff in the Gantry. Well, there is Luke, Crystal and Reenie. I haven't talked about Crystal and Reenie because I would get no sympathy what so ever if you folks ever saw them. They are both very attractive young ladies, both with a great sense of humor, mixed in with compassion for all their patients. Next week I will try and get a picture of the entire group. Obviously, they know me very well, you might say intimately!!!

Golf for the day was fine...just a little cooler than yesterday, not much but a little. My heavy heart was repaired a little, but still has a crack in it. Ray and Gary won the front side, we won the back side, and they won the overall. Last chance tomorrow to fix my cracked heart. We will be playing the final day at North Hampton, it's supposed to be the most difficult of the three. Scores today will not be mentioned as all four players stunk. No, maybe worse than that, but I can't come up with a worse word. I know you're not going to believe this, but I sprained my left wrist getting out of the car today....it didn't hurt too bad at impact, but definitely effected my follow through and overall game.

Mike was so concerned about my injury that it effected his game also. Don't ask me where I come up with these things, they just come out. On the way home we stopped to get some ice cream.

After arriving home all four hit the sack. I only took a short nap, I believe I'm wearing these old men out. In fact, as I'm writing now, two of the four are still asleep.

Just to report on all the wonderful items Beverly, Brenda and Susan sent down. Half the peanut brittle is gone, half the banana bread is gone. Only half of one coconut pie is left of the two sent. All the brownies are gone...we took them to the golf course. I believe these guys are going to leave me food-less when they leave.

Dinner tonight is still up in the air....either oysters at the oyster shack or Baxter's....not sure yet. Went to Baxter's and had a great time. The three of them had the steak sandwich that is awesome....having a toned body now, I just had soup and a salad. They met everyone, the owner, Ethan and even an old friend of Mikes was there...simper fi....that's what I call him because Al is an ex-marine.

OK folks, I want you to note and duly record this next bit of very important information. As you know, I have been a doctor, pastor, and senator before....now I have decided to become an attorney (sorry Stan), and here is the reason why. Mike purchased this beautiful place a year ago and completely remodeled it, then had his daughter decorate it to the nines, but Mike and Donna have spent a small amount of time here. I have spent more time here than Mike. As an attorney now, I am declaring squatters rights and have taken over ownership of this stately location and beautiful home. With one exception, Mike has to continue to pay the taxes and any other neighborhood dues that are required. DONE!

My son leaves for Russia today on a business trip....wow. Please keep him in your prayers. Most of you reading this can probably still remember the cold war with Russia when you were in high school, I can. I'm sure it will be a wonderful trip and highly educational. I love you son, have a great trip.

It's late, even past my normal bedtime......**Good night everyone.**

July 28, 2012 (Saturday) **We Won!**

Rejoice my heart, rejoice, I believe that's a biblical statement from lst John, but not sure, I'll have to check with John Cook on that ....yes we won today!!! It was nip and tuck today but Mike birdied the 17th hole which ended up winning it for us (we were four shots down at the time, what a comeback)...showing nice guys don't finish last. Here's the interesting thing, we won with both of us having sprained ankles and me having a sprained wrist. I got the people at the treatment center to tape my wrist and that got me through this final round. After 14 or 15 holes I had already drawn up a For Sale sign for my clubs and numerous pairs of golf shoes. Mike got me pumped up and with his birdie and we pulled it out... we did it!!!

Help me out, when you get a moment, please go out and buy Ray and Gary a sympathy card, maybe it will pick them up a bit. During our round, we stopped and got the cart girl to take a picture of the four of us....after she took the picture, she asked if she could have one with me and of course, I gave in and let her do it. Pictures will follow....

Stopped by the Ice Cream place and I thought Ray was going to eat all the ice cream they had. Got home and put our bathing suits on and went for a swim....the water felt awesome. Of course I got all the attention with my new white speedo swim suit. Gary didn't go and Ray and Mike were so jealous of my terrific looking speedo. Maybe when I get home the Sunday school class will have a cookout and swim party....you think? I think not!!!

Had a great dinner tonight. We went to Brett's on the Waterway. While we were there Ray gave us a health talk and lesson. These were his wise comments....Don't get the grouper, because it's on rice which has starch which is not good for you. It's ok to eat things like cookies, peanut brittle, coconut cream pie, brownies and banana nut bread, but don't eat the grouper because it's on rice with all that starch. So there you go folk's .....A short lesson for your health. *"Why do I feel I just had a conversation with Yogi Berra?"* By-the-way, Gary, Mike and I had one brownie each, Ray ate the rest of them...He will say he didn't, but he did.

It has really been nice having these guys down to my place this week, we have had a lot of fun and many, many laughs. More importantly, I got to know Ray and Mike a little better than I had in the past and they both are quality guys. They all will be missed when they leave in the morning. (Not really, but I want them to think that!)

Only one bad thing, they brought me all this food from Beverly, Brenda and Susan which was wonderful, but they ate it all.....hopefully I will be able to make it through the next two weeks and not starve to death.

Thank goodness for Baxter's!!!

Wow, almost 10 pm....**Good night everyone.**

Chapter 17

A Journey With Me

Week 7

<u>July 29, 2012 (Sunday)</u> **God Bless You All**

Well the boys are packing up and getting ready to go. I cooked bacon and egg sandwiches for everyone so they would not have to stop on the way. Of course, Ray wanted the last piece of banana nut bread with his sandwich...Joan (Ray's wife), what is your grocery bill each month? It must be a fortune, or at least a small fortune. Unreal, can't believe how quiet it is in the condo!

Only TEN more treatments left. (Find it hard to believe I've already had 29 treatments) I honestly feel the time has gone by pretty fast, but at my age, time seems to fly. It seems like only yesterday I was in high school. Maybe it's just my mind playing tricks on me. Of course my motto has always been "Growing old is mandatory, growing up is optional, and I choose not to" Staying young is so much more fun, and it makes dealing with life's ups and downs so much easier. Don't you think?

Wanted to take this opportunity to thank Sam and Suzanne Lilly for the very nice card they sent me. You don't realize how much I appreciate it, and what it means to me. Other than the circular fan in the Sunday school class, I'm probably Sam's only other fan....one funny man and a great couple. Thanks guys for your help.

Today is cleanup day....the boys left a mess. Four sets of sheets to wash and beds to make up...towels and wash cloths, including beach towels. Trash to take out, dishes to wash and put away. I bet I could make someone a good wife one of these days.....not!

Got a call from George Breece today and George Crumbley walked by George and said hello to me also....isn't Mr. Crumbley the head pastor at Highland Presbyterian Church now? Sorry Ernie. George Breece, Frank Maynard, and Gary and I did everything together growing up. Believe it or not, all four of us took piano lessons from a lady named Mrs. Cook when we were in elementary school. As I reflect back on that, I really feel sorry for that woman. However, to this day I can still play a song or two that I learned for recital. Again, really do feel sorry for that poor woman....don't you? Mrs. Cook did let Gary and me take for free.....we did have to buy the sheet music however, must have at least been about a dime a sheet or less, and can't remember.

OK, let's get this cleared up right now and eliminate any misunderstanding that might have taken place by any of my Sunday school fellow (male) friends. Someone from the Sunday school class emailed me and told me that I had really stepped on my own toes. None of the guys had any sympathy for me any more after seeing the picture of me with the cart girl. Come on guys, has no one ever heard of photo Shoppe....you can do anything magical with a computer now. I did love Jay's comments however, at least once I caught on. Thanks Jay. You and Stafford are a hoot, and I'll never forget the night you two and David and Diane pulled that trick on me at Baxter's.

Several people have asked, Jerry how do you know if that Proton stuff is working? Very good question. When I leave here I will receive orders to have a PSA test done again in Fayetteville after three months. A normal PSA test is 1 or less, or at least that is ideal, I'm told. When I came to Amelia Island, my PSA was 7.2 and I had a Gleason score of 6. The 7.2 is not good at all, the Gleason score of 6 is very good. Everyone here in Jacksonville is very positive and quite frankly, I'm not really worried at all....well, just a little.

I don't know how much longer this journal will continue. I will say this, I have had a blast writing it, but more importantly getting the emails from everyone and their comments brought me so many laughs. I believe it has been somewhat funny, somewhat inspirational and hopefully informative about Proton Treatment. It has probably brought a laugh and a tear, possibly? But my main goal was to show that cancer is not the end, and how much a positive attitude can go towards healing (or anything else as far as that is concerned)....with God's help that is!

My family and friends have come and gone....I'm on my own now (and I think that's good in that it gives me time to reflect on everything that has happened over the last 8 weeks), but want to express what strong feelings I have for each and every one of you. My heart is bursting with pride knowing that so many wonderful people care, not just for me, but many, many others. You see it with Operation Inasmuch, you see it with what our class does for others, here and overseas. There are so many of you that continue to help at every level, big or small, and right down to the smallest gift, they are all appreciated. I only pray that I have shown my appreciation to all of you in some small way. Not only for just this little bout with cancer, but for what all of have you done for me and my family over the last year...! God bless you all!

Folks, as I typed the previous paragraph, I must admit several tears of joy fell down my cheeks (I get emotional at ground clearings for new 7-11 stores)....but I really want to end on a very positive note, so here it is.... I just read an email from my buddy Frank Upchurch, and I love him to death, and this is the type of quality person he is. He said that the men in the Sunday school class were raising money to put together a mission trip, so they could come down and help me with the cart girl situation....now how thoughtful is that. He also said further details would follow. Just as a reminder to everyone......photo Shoppe, George Holden, please explain what that means to everyone please.

I'm tired and ready to get this treatment over.....**Good night everyone.**

<u>July 30, 2012 (Monday)</u> **A Call from Afghanistan, and August 10th**

Failed to mention in yesterday's journal the man I saw at Baxter's last night. It was a very small crowd and this man came in and took some napkins and started writing on them. When Matt went over to serve him, the man handed him the napkins. He had written his order on them. I spoke to Matt later and asked what that was all about. He said the man could not speak or hear. When Matt brought him his order, it was 5 boxes of food to go. I can only imagine, he has a wife and 3 children. Matt says he speaks to people by using his phone and showing them a text. Sure wish I had met him, hopefully he will come back in while I'm there before I leave. I'd love to learn more about him.

Today's treatment was a little different. When I got out of the shower this morning, I realized my markings were gone. They must have come off in the pool this weekend. The markings are how they line me up in my body cast

153

before they shoot the Proton. A couple of big X's on my hips. Making a joke out of it, they said it looked like I may have to start over.....funny...not. (On top of that, I told them I'll do the funny stuff) I did have to have a couple CAT scans to line up with the old film so they could be sure they were shooting in the right direction...no big deal really. Starting over would not even been an option!

Started back walking yesterday and I honestly believe I'm getting close to the five mile mark. (Look out Stan....the only thing about being in second is the view is always the same) Yesterday and today's walk was nice and getting easier by the day. Did not walk when the boys were here for golf, simply because of the golf and the heat we all endured during the day.
For those of you that were in high school with me, I wanted to let you know that I get quite a few emails from Ginger Bobbitt. She has a nice looking family and her son is serving our country....he flies some type of aircraft I believe. Just a little information to pass on.

Tell me my day wasn't just made today. I just received a phone call from Jon Cook in Afghanistan, wishing me well, and asking me to set up a twin match with Gary in early September. He is over in Afghanistan fighting for our country and takes time to call me to see how I'm doing...unreal. Jon and Josh are twins of John and Gaye Cook, pastor at our church. After playing golf with them the first time, the Sunday School class ask me what I thought of them. I said, they are good looking, great personalities, and excellent golfers and remind me so much of Gary and me.....well, me anyway. They call Gary Santa, and me Job. Too long a story to tell where those names come from. Made my day Jon!!!!

I don't know how your day can be made twice in one day, but it can. Listen to this. I use a devotional book

154

named Jesus Calling, by Sarah Young. Well, I just got an email from Susan saying to look at what it says on August 10 (August 10 is the day of my last treatment). The heading on August 10th is "Relax in my Healing", pretty cool, huh? Jon, one minute, "Relax in my Healing" the next minute. Do we have an awesome God or what?

Educational time.....radiation starts killing the minute it enters your body and kills until it leaves your body....Proton treatment enters your body and does not kill until it reaches your tattooed tumor and then explodes and stops there, not going any further in your body. By-the-way that is a layman's explanation. Although, I did play a doctor on TV.

Dinner at Baxter's, a healthy Philly Cheese sandwich with fries. Watching my weight you know. I have to be able to fit in that body cast they put me in each morning. It's really not a big deal folks.....the cast that is. Ethan was there and we picked at each other for about an hour, but had fun. Small crown again tonight. I preform so much better in front of a crowd.

Good night everyone....after tomorrow, only 8 more left. Hope each of you had as wonderful a day as I did, and may tomorrow be even better.

July 31, 2012 (Tuesday) **Prayers for Caden, Kim and Willie**

Treatment went well, and today was my day (this week) to see the doctor. Blood pressure high, a little, and weight 175. Met with Barbara the nurse first. I like Barbara and Tracey a lot, Barbara is a diabetic, I found out today and she wears a pump for her insulin. The pump sure hasn't affected her attractiveness. She and Tracey are both fun to be around. Didn't get home until almost lunch time so went out and got a chicken salad sandwich. I did meet another patient today who sings in a gospel group. I looked them up on the internet and they are awesome....for a special treat, look this up www.The3AMMovement.Squarespace.com (These guys are terrific) I asked if they needed another person for the group and he politely said, no thank you. I guess singing is out, the audition with him went well I thought....oh well. Believe it or not, they sound a little like the Boys to Men group.....great harmony.

Need to make a request of everyone....this Friday my grandson (Caden Scottie Williams) goes in for a heart checkup. He was born with a small defect that hopefully he will outgrow, but I would appreciate everyone remembering him this Friday, his mother Kim (my daughter) also. My second request is for my dear friend Willie. This Thursday she is going to have back surgery for pain she has been experiencing for quite some time now. She and John, I'm sure, would appreciate it. Thanks everyone. It's a beautiful overcast day and now its walk time. Made it just in time, when I got home it started raining cats and dogs...good timing.

Little trivia here....how many of you are familiar with the term, the Freedom Bird? That's what my friend (Frank) and other troops called the plane that was taking them out of Vietnam at the end of their tour there. My Freedom Bird is on its way to pick me up from here. Unfortunately, mine is a Freedom Car that will be taking me home, but it will feel like the Freedom Bird. Will miss all the fine people I have met here, but there is just no place like home.

Dinner at Baxter's tonight was outstanding. Met another new couple and they were interesting. The interesting part was they both were on their second marriages. One had 4 children and the other had 3 when they got married....can you imagine, 7 children in the house at once. Well they have been married for quite some time....you got to know that took a lot of work. Of course Ethan was there being his usual charming self. I had just a salad with shrimp.

This next paragraph may shock the world.....I stayed up until after 11:45 pm watching gymnastics win the gold. Those girls (the fab five, they were called) were awesome. I kept saying, I'll go just as soon as the next event was over......and then saying that again. Tomorrow is going to be a very long day.

USA, USA, USA.........**Good night everyone.**

August 1, 2012 (Wednesday) **Chris Cammack will always be my All-American**

The drive in this morning was exceptionally beautiful...there are rivers everywhere, in fact, Jacksonville is known as the city of rivers. One of the things I noticed this morning was how beautiful the marsh areas are. They honestly look like someone paid special attention to plant them just where they are, so uniform and such. Then it hit me....someone did plant them, as well as, all the other beauty on this great earth.

Treatment went well...only 7 more left. Met a couple this morning that were from Atlanta and they were just checking out this Proton thing. He (Dick) asked me a ton of questions and I was very confident in the fact that I believe this type of treatment has been a blessing to prostate cancer and many others.

I also found out that Emory University in Atlanta is in the process of building a facility, but it's about three years off. Also found out they are starting to treat some forms of breast cancer with this Proton....who knows where it will end.

Got an email from Greg telling me my buddy Chris is home from his surgery. Chris will always be my All-American...which he was, two or three years at NC State. I believe he still holds the highest batting average ever at State. Everyone keep him in your prayers.

Another couple that I have met while here is Norman and Barbara Barber. They were both widowed and when they started dating, Barbara told Norman that she doubted she would ever marry him...he asked why? Her response was I don't want to be called Barbara Barber the rest of my life. It does sound just a little strange, but guess what she will be called the rest of her life....you got it, Barbara Barber. They both are very nice and more importantly, they are big UGA fans...go dawgs.

Had a great walk and realized how much easier it is getting each day. Each day I try to extend my length a little longer....who knows, I may walk home. No, I couldn't do that...who would carry my clothes and golf clubs.

Drove to downtown Fernandina Beach this evening just to walk around a little. By the way, Frank and I stopped by the place we had the cigar and thanked Joe for setting up the golf at Amelia National....nice guy. That may be as nice a course as I have ever played. There are a lot of beautiful old buildings downtown, as well as, a lot of tourist. Of course, I'm a regular here.

Got back home and had the left over spaghetti from when Ray, Gary and Mike were here. I don't know why, but why does the sauce seem to taste better the second time you have it. I can't wait until the third time. Watched our USA team a bit and then hit the sack. Only 7 more treatments left....that's almost hard to believe.

Good night everyone.

<u>August 2, 2012 (Thursday)</u> **Scottie is looking down with a Smile**

At treatment today I saw a lot of new faces. Wondered what was going on and as it turned out, these guys were here for their 5 year checkups. I talked with several of them to get a little information on how they were doing. The highest PSA test for any of them was less than 1, that's remarkable. I also did not talk with anyone that had any side effects at all. I left the treatment center thinking....wow, these men have really confirmed my thinking that I have been led to the best treatment for prostate cancer. I know there are medical reasons for choosing another alternative, but if you qualify, why would you not choose this method over surgery or some other alternative.

You know, I am so glad I grew up when I did. It was a simple life without a lot of issues and everyday was spent at the Honeycutt rec. center. You played all day and were not considered dirty until you had at least two rings around your neck. Growing up in Fayetteville was fun, Junior high school, Fayetteville Senior High School (and students respected the adults), sports, friends and no cares in the world....it was a blast. Today, it's not quite that way....there are way too many issues and distractions. I don't particularly care for my age, but have sure had a wonderful life.

Went to the grocery store this evening and received a call from my daughter while I was there. Kim is involved in a parent visitation situation in court today and needless to say, I was concerned over the outcome. I have always told Keith and Kim, "Don't ever let them see your Sweat". Well, the outcome was awesome. The remarkable thing was, after the court time was over, the judge came up to Kim and said, "You are the Rock of Gibraltar". I am so proud of her I don't know what to do.

As mentioned earlier, I was in the grocery store, and the first thing I did after the phone call was visit the Kleenex department....I am such a wimp. Now, if we can get through this issue in the morning with Caden's heart, it will be a great weekend...Please pray for Caden. I've known two women personally that had to raise children as a single parent. It's got to be tough!!! The reason for the previous paragraph was just to point out how more difficult it must be today. Just inflation alone hits you upside the head like a two by four (child care for example). Kim has had some major difficulties as a single mom (as most do), but I am as proud of her as any parent could ever be of their child. I also know Scottie is looking down at her with a great deal of pride and one big smile. You know, being a parent is tough enough, being a single parent even much more difficult.

  John Dunigan gave me a book that I believe I still haven't returned to him. In it, there was a statement made about a parent that was really worried about his children when he was away from home. This man came up to him and said, why are you worried....they are not your kids...they are God's children. I'm guessing that says volumes...don't you.
Finished my shopping, and went home and had a great dinner. Seafood, can you imagine! Here's what I can't imagine....ONLY 6 TREATMENTS LEFT!!!!!

It's late....**Good night everyone.**

August 3, 2012 (Friday) **Thank you Lord for Taking Care of Caden**

Treatment went well....only bad thing today was having to say goodbye to some friends from Duluth Ga....the

Barbers. Good people, and who knows, may run into them again at a Georgia Football game...you never know. I also met another fella from Charlotte, N.C., he was here for a 5 year checkup and as I questioned him....his response was, doing great, no side effects what so ever. Love this stuff!

Got home and had a call from Kim telling me about Caden's doctor's appointment this morning to check out his heart. Kim said it went perfectly and he does not have to go back until a year later....what great news! While walking on the beach, I kept saying, thank You Lord, thank You Lord for taking care of Caden for me since I couldn't be there to get him through this heart thing. I also got to thinking about something my mother (Mrs. Barnhill) always told me. She would say... "God answers all prayer, you just may not like all His answers, such as no and later, but he definitely answers all prayer." What a great walk it was!

At the conclusion of my walk, I decided to try the ocean for a bit to help me cool down, I walk at a torrid pace. Be aware that I'm not a great swimmer and have a great deal of respect for any body of water, especially the ocean. As I was walking out a little deeper a wave hit me like a ton of bricks. It actually knocked me down and almost knocked the breath out of me. I don't believe I was ever hit that hard playing football. Didn't want any more of that....As Henry said to Janet one night....count me doubtful on going back into the water. As I was sitting under an umbrella resting from the hit I had just received I saw two couples walking out to the beach.

I have seen white people, and I have seen white people, these two couples were white on white. At one point, I thought one of the women had on a pair of white hose...now folks...I am not embellishing at all here. They laid out their towels and laid down.....I would have loved to run into them around 5 or 6 o'clock. I bet the only place I could have found them was in the emergency room.

Got home and took a great nap...woke up and did a little ironing, cleaning and such, then showered, shaved and got ready to go to

Baxter's. As usual, Ethan was there and a few others I knew, but kind of quiet crowd. Ethan is one funny guy....going to miss him when I leave. He sure has brought a lot of laughs and smiles to my face.

Don't know what I'm going to do this weekend, as you may be aware or not, it is my last weekend on Amelia!!!!!!!! May go to Walmart and get a 3 day fishing license and try and catch a whale or something like that. It really doesn't matter if you catch anything or not, it's a great way to pass some time while on the beach. Regardless, I hope I have better luck than Bobby and I have had at Kure Beach over the years. I once told Bobby, I don't believe the Bible was right on that sea thing....I just can't believe God put any fish in it, and if he did, he didn't put any at Kure Beach.

Folks, need your help....I was talking with Bob this morning (not to be confused with BOB!), he gets on the treatment table just before me. We were talking about the fact that he was about to become a grandparent for the first time. His kids will not tell anyone what the name is going to be, or whether it's going to be a girl or boy. He was telling me about an old wives tale which I have never heard before. You hold a string and pen or needle over a mothers belly and depending on which way it leans, will determine if it's a boy or girl......that's where I need the help, does the left or right determine if it's a boy? Anyone know, or has Bob totally lost his mind from the treatments here? It appears I have! I spent the rest of the morning telling him about Grace, Luke and Caden.....

As you can probably tell from this writing....its late folks....**Good night everyone.**

<u>August 4, 2012 (Saturday)</u> **Bobby, where have all the Fish gone?**

No BOB today. Had a nice breakfast and headed to Walmart to check out the fishing gear and check on a three day fishing license.

Getting someone to help you in Walmart is like pulling eye teeth, maybe worse. I would go up to other customers and say "are you a fisherman?" If there response was yes, I would start drilling them with questions on how to catch a nice flounder....my favorite fish to eat, plus grouper. I got all types of ideas on what type of rig to put together and the customers were very helpful. Once I had all my fish hunting supplies and what type of rig to use I went to the counter to pay. Guess what....no one there. I finally had to go to the front of the store and ask the manager if he wanted to sell something today, if so, I will be waiting at the sports counter. Didn't have to wait much longer after that.

One of the strange things about getting help from the customers....the one that helped me the most could have been a young Fred Ritter, looked like him quite a bit, including the visor.
Look cut fish, here I come. I figured if I just caught two fish, each weighing two pounds each....I would be paying about $25 per pound. Are they not cheaper than that at Harris Teeter...I'm going to check that out?

Fished for about an hour and never even got a nibble, it

also started to rain....Bobby, I don't believe there are any fish down here either....I know there are none at Kure Beach....are we sure that Bible thing is correct. I just don't believe Noah put any fish on the Ark.

Got home, had a nice sandwich for lunch...nap time.

Spent most of the day watching the Olympics on TV. Finished up the spaghetti that was left over and got to bed early. I'm going to try that fishing thing in the morning I guess.

Good night everyone.

Chapter 18

A Journey With Me

Week 8

<u>August 5, 2012 (Sunday)</u> **Great Grandmother Rich, What a Woman!**

They say the most important meal of the day is breakfast....not sure who they are, but that's what they say. Went to the store and got some bacon, and a cantaloupe. I fixed bacon, eggs, grits, and toast with cantaloupe for dessert. The only thing missing was homemade biscuits with molasses. Put a little churned butter on the molasses and sop it up with your biscuit and you're in heaven.

While eating this morning I got to thinking about those rings around the neck and a big breakfast. When Gary and I were young (6,7or 8) mother (Mrs. Barnhill) would take us to Garland, N.C. for a couple of weeks or maybe more. She did this to give herself a break I'm sure. Garland is where the most incredible woman in the world lived. My Grandmother Rich. She lived to be 102 and had eleven children (a Sunday school is named after her in the little Baptist Church there) She buried most of children which was sad. On her farm in Garland she raised tobacco. She had a very mean cow, lots of chickens and who knows what else. We had some great cousins there....at one of their houses, they had goats and we would chase them and try to ride them. You talk about ring around the neck!! We never worked in tobacco but got to ride in the sled that the mule pulled as they put the tobacco in it....her home had no electricity, or running water. The most trouble we got into was locking a cousin in the outhouse....I'm not sure which one. (And yes, I have used a Sears catalog). There was no grass to cut...you would sweep the yard.

 When we needed to get rid of those rings, grandmother would fill up the tub on the back porch and clean us up. I can't remember even if the water was warm, she may have warmed it up a bit on her wood stove in the kitchen. In the kitchen was also the fly paper. It sure kept the flies off the food. I can also remember on a few occasions, helping her churn butter, the old fashion way. I can't remember what level of education she achieved, but it doesn't matter, she was one intelligent woman. When she attended school, they didn't have paper to write on, she would write on a slate of some type.

 This woman was always respected by her children and grandchildren....somewhat revered, and she deserved it. As I grew older and got married and moved away, I did not get to see her that often, maybe once or twice a year, or at a family reunion. However, when I did see her, I would always give her a big hug and tell her how much I enjoyed hugging big breasted women....for some reason, she would always get a kick out of it (and I did this until she was way into her 90's, maybe 100's), and it always brought a beautiful smile to her beautiful face. I'm probably the only one that could have gotten away with that. In fact, I am sure of that!

 She did love her grandchildren (Gary and I were always special to her I felt), don't even know how many she had, but family reunions were big. Does anyone ever have those anymore? Few do, and that's sad also. See all the information you can get by eating a good breakfast and thinking about rings around your neck, and aren't all grandmothers and nana's wonderful?

After lunch, I went back to the sea and gave it another try, same result. Speaking of fishing, my friend Greg, noticing an interest I've acquired in fishing sent me a great fish quote...."Give a man a fish and he will eat all day, teach a man to fish, and he will sit in a boat and drink beer all day" Thanks Greg for that bit of information...! By-the-way, that fish per pound right now stands at $100. A pound. I know Harris Teeter is cheaper that that!

Went to Baxter's tonight and had a wonderful dinner. Pineapple Grouper...it was outstanding (Thanks Sam and Suzanne). Several of my new found friends were there also. It was good to see them all and I shared with them that this was my last week here on the Island. Of course, they were all upset, a few cried and a few applauded.....all kidding aside, these are some wonderful people that I have met here and they all will be missed.

As I told some of them tonight, I dreaded the fact that I had to come here for so long, and now, I hate to say goodbye to them. They will all be missed.

Wow, it's almost 9:30....**Good night everyone.**

August 6, 2012 (Monday) **The fine Mayor, Billy Bob**

Weird day...my appointment was to be at 8:56 this morning. When I arrived from my 40 minute drive a posting showed the gantry was down. After waiting some time and drinking my water a posting came up, gantry will be down 360 minutes I headed back to Amelia and asked that they call me when it's my turn. On the way back home they called and said it would be around noon. I headed back around 11 only to find out the gantry was still down. As it turned out, I finally got my treatment around 3:45. Was I upset...no way! I have been so fortunate throughout 34 treatments, not one problem. With only 4 treatments left why get upset. By the way, the gantry is what the treatment room is called and I later found out the mother board went down closing all three gantries. Did meet some newcomers there for their first day, they were not taking the situation very well....oh well. With all the water I drank today for treatments and rescheduling, I believe I set a world record for quick stops on the way home. Why do they not put bathrooms in automobiles? Somehow build them into the steering wheel....I guess not.

I heard from my high powered attorney today concerning my speeding ticket I received coming down here. Here is how it went. The Mayor of this little town, Billy Bob, called Jason (my attorney) and asked how he could help. The mayor told Jason (Heather's husband) to call the police chief, Billy Bob Jr. and tell him of my situation. Billy Bob Jr. sent him an email telling him he would get it reduced if he would send a letter telling him of my circumstances. I love this country....justice for all. Can you believe this little town receives either 2 or 3 million dollars a year on tickets? I wonder what size house Billy Bob and his son live in anyway. I bet they have some big tractors. I thought for a while I might have to call in my other high powered attorney Stan from Roanoke, I know personally he has spent some time on the farm. By the way, this is not a put down of people in the country or farmers.

They are the hardest working people in the world as far as I am concerned. I just believe these people have a racket going on in South Georgia. I will be driving with caution while going through Georgia. Thanks Jason, I really do understand why Gary said he would marry you if Heather didn't.

Oh well, what do I care...I only have 4 more treatments left. I know this sounds crazy, but I am really going to miss these people here. Those at the treatment center and here on the Island. They all have gone overboard to see that my stay has been as pleasant as it could be.

Went to Baxter's to visit with my friends Ethan and Al, came home and had some left overs and then to bed. It was definitely a long day with all the trips to Jacksonville.

Good night Mrs. Calabash, where ever you are....and thanks Jimmy Durante. I hope I got that right!!!!

Good night everyone.

<u>August 7, 2012 (Tuesday)</u> **How Can I Thank all the People?**

Treatment was not uncomfortable at all today....do not know why, but everything went well. I did learn that Thursday when I see the doctor I will have some blood work done which will give me some type of indication as to how the treatments are working. Part of the blood work will be a PSA examine. When the treatments started, my PSA was over 7 and we would like to get it down to 1 or less....I guess we will see.

After getting back I started what I called my prep day. (Preparing to go home) I did a little cleaning. I started to do a very little packing. Went to the beach for a bit but the sun kept going behind clouds. Went to the Harris Teeter down here to get a few things for dinner. Called Ethan to have him set up my final round of golf at Amelia National....I do love that golf course. I am going to play with Matt, one of the employees at Baxter's.

Dinner time.....I know Kirby doesn't believe me, but here is what I had for dinner. Fried Chicken, rice and gravy, Corn on the cob, homemade cold slaw. Corn bread (Larry Sessoms makes the best corn bread I've ever had).

The two things missing were fried okra, and butter beans. Everything was very good and the chicken would have been even better if I had had my iron skillet with me. By the way Mr. Bill Kirby, this was not take out from Baxter's.

It really has been a very quiet, beautiful, uneventful day, but a day I have enjoyed. Basically the only concern I've had today is how I'm going to wrap this writing thing up, and bring everything to an end. Also, how can I thank all the people who have visited, phoned, emailed, sent things, cooked things.....the list goes on and on. Like the call I received from Afghanistan. The only other major concern is overlooking thanking someone, I pray that doesn't happen.

ONLY 3 TREATMENTS LEFT!!!!!!!!!!!!!!

Good night everyone.....

<u>August 8, 2012 (Wednesday)</u> **"Immortal Memory"**

Got to see my little buddy Easton this morning. He is the 23 month old that is being treated for a tumor they have already removed from his brain. His Nana said they are doing the Proton just to be sure everything is gone for good. Met a fellow named Mike this morning. His last day for treatment is also this Friday. Mike is a member of the TPC, at Sawgrass. Too bad I didn't get to meet him earlier. Next month, he and his sons are going to Scotland to play. Scottie and I had a wonderful time in Scotland 11 years ago. She has a cousin that is from Barrhead Scotland. He was able to get me on Royal

Troon once while we were there. Her cousin is quite the artist. To see some of his work, he can be found at www.chaskelly.com.

To me, his best work is a piece I have in my home which is a tribute to Robert Burns called "Immortal Memory."

I found out that we, as patients were able to play the TPC.....for the low price of $175.....which is their summer rate. I'm not sure if I would pay that to play Augusta National....well maybe once.

Got home and headed to the golf course. I called my friend Ethan the other day and asked him to get me on Amelia National one more time...he said, you know

Wilson, you are becoming a pain in the butt. That's a north easterners way of saying he likes you. Playing with Matt who works at Baxter's and really looking forward to playing that golf course. It reminds me a lot of Forest Creek. Chris Cammack took Gary and me over to Forest Creek and it is nice on nice, really first class. Sure hope my Friend Chris is doing OK! Continue to keep him in your prayers please.
We played and enjoyed this fabulous course one more time. It was overcast making it a little cooler. I played OK, but had fun. The nice thing about playing golf in Florida this time of year is, if you can stand the heat, it's like you are the only one on the course, no delay in play what so ever.

Yummy dinner, just an old fashion hamburger, with cold slaw, mustard and a big slice of onion, and chips. Maybe I should open a hamburger, hot dog stand in Fayetteville and call it Hot Diggity Dog, you think that may work?

After tomorrow I will have one more treatment, a total of 39. The people here have been an absolute delight...

everyone. Somewhat of a conclusion....this will be the last blog or journal posting I will do until I receive the results of this treatment. I have enjoyed writing about this journey and hopefully some of you have enjoyed reading it. I have tried to be honest most of the time, as well as, add a little humor which, is as far as I am concerned, the real spice of life. Cancer is not something to make fun of, but one's attitude is so important during the treatment process. Thanks to all of you who have taken your time to read my silliness, all the characters mentioned in this blog are fictional and not to be confused with any one from Fayetteville or Amelia Island.

Good night everyone....and may God Bless you. May good health follow you and hopefully your life will never be touched by cancer.

Chapter 19

The Final Chapter (Blog)

Thanksgiving has come and gone and Christmas is just a few days away. I felt it would be a good time to put together the final chapter with my thoughts on this little journey called prostate cancer. Quite frankly, I do have so many things to be thankful for, and the results of the treatment in Florida at the University Of Florida Proton Treatment Center is just one of them.

The difficult part of writing this final chapter is where do I begin? First and foremost, I want to thank all the people that kept me in their prayers and thoughts. I am a firm believer in prayer, and the power of prayer. There is no doubt in my mind that God hears and answers them all. Thank you God!

I also want to thank the Pleasants for providing me a beautiful place to stay for the eight weeks I was in Florida. All the money in the world could not repay your generosity and you both will always have a special place in my heart, especially since Mike made that birdie on the 17thhole to carry us on to victory. I also want to thank all of you who visited and or called or sent cards and gifts and care packages while I was in Florida. Each visit was special, each card was read with enthusiasm, and each phone call was received with an open heart and love.

Well, almost all of them! The night I received the call from the mafia in Chicago got my blood pressure up quite a bit. However, so much laughter has happened just recalling the prank David, Diane, Jay and Stafford played on me. I'm sure I deserved it. Each gift and care package was received as being golden and enjoyed by me and others that were visiting me. Ray sure got his fair share.

 I also want to thank Bill Kirby for running my silliness on his blog. I have received so many remarks (and some of them were good) from people that said how much they enjoyed reading the blog. One person in particular said he felt like he was involved in a soap opera…he couldn't wait to read the next day's blog!

The progress from the treatment in Florida continues to improve. I started out with a PSA of 7.4, when I left Florida the results were 3.4 and then it went to 1.9. It is currently at a wonderful 0.68 which is fine. The most amazing thing about the treatment is I have had no side effects what so ever. This is a wonderful thing, especially when I hear some of the horrible stories of others who went in a different direction.

When I first started tracking my PSA with my local doctor, he said he was concerned…so was I. No one at any time wants to hear the word cancer, and having been through it once…I surly didn't. We decided to go to Duke for further test and a biopsy. Well the biopsy was positive, with a Gleason score of $3 + 3 = 6$. Cancer was found in 6 of the 12 cores they removed. Now, what do I do? Each doctor I spoke with said the decision for treatment was my decision. I only finished two years of medical school and Prostate cancer was covered only in the third year. Each doctor I spoke with was leaning towards their way (which I understand), but they all continued to say the decision was mine. After much research, reading and personally talking with patients that had been through the process,

I decided on Proton treatments. Mainly because of a fluke one day when my sister Beverly was doing someone's hair did I hear about the Proton Treatment in Jacksonville, Florida. Well as mentioned several times, I am very happy with the treatment and especially the results...who wouldn't be. However, I received a letter the other day from my urologist here in Fayetteville that I have been seeing for some time. He has done an excellent job and relieved me from a lot of pain with kidney stones and such, as well as other issues I have had over the years. However, he was not pleased that I chose to go to Florida for the treatments. His letter said he had read of my treatments in the paper and because I had chosen to not use him, he asked that I please come by and get my records for I was no longer a patient of his...I had been fired, was my guess. Well good doctor, thanks for all you have done in the past, you are truly as asset to this community and city.

I do hope you understand it was not an easy decision, and one that was made with much thought and prayer. I thought doctors had to take some type of oath...I guess not! If there is a urologist who might by chance be reading this blog, and is taking new patients, I would love to hear from you and your staff to set up an appointment...I have been fired, and probably without any severance pay.

Keith ramrodded a welcome home party with the help of Beverly, Gary and Brenda. It has to fall in the top five events I've experienced in my life. Not the party itself, but rather the number of people that took time out of their lives to brighten mine. Thank you, thank you, thank you, each and every one of you. My aunts were there, even Pauline drove down from Morehead, NC.

175

My dear friend that cut my son's hair for the first time over 40 years ago was there, Dewey and Beverly from Greensboro. Many of my Sunday school class members were there and as we all know, they are the finest people in the world. There were also classmates and many other friends. Letters from those that could not attend saying how much they hated to miss it.

One of my favorite letters was from an old competitor from High School days from Rocky Mount. Danny Talbot, in my mind one of the finest, if not the best, all-around athletes to ever come out of the state of NC…Danny has also had some issues with cancer, but I understand he is doing very well now. Keith's comments were very funny and MC, and the letter Bill Kirby wrote still brings a tear to my eye even as I write this final chapter…thanks Bill. Of course the highlight was the note I received from the Golf Commissioner inviting me to join the PGA tour. Sure wish I had the talent to do that, but the people at eh Florida Proton center said they did not have the medicine strong enough to fix my golf game! Oh well, maybe in another life.

I have a friend here in Fayetteville that I play golf with occasionally. The other day she told me her new priorities were…God, Family, and Golf. I loved it. My new priorities are God, Family, Friends, Golf, Everything else, and then Urologist.

Christ said, "And the greatest of these is love". I have nothing but love in my heart for all those who helped and encouraged me during this process, and I might add unconditional love. May God bless you all and grant you wonderful health throughout your life.

Conclusion:

One of the nicest surprises at the welcome home party, was the attendance of three of my aunts, Leona "Sasser" Barnhill, Joanne McCormick and Pauline Long. My aunt Pauline, who passed away this year, traveled all the way from Morehead City, NC. Pauline could cook the best fried shrimp I have ever had in my life, along with her delicious cold slaw and Strawberry cake.

They all (emails and letters) meant so much to me. They all renewed my faith and gave me much encouragement. These emails are not listed in any type of order or date received, just randomly picked from many, many emails of encouragement.

PS: Each email may not be complete as it was sent. I have modified some and of course, embellished most! The following pages will consist of a few of the many emails I received, and some letters which were read at the Welcome Home Party. I was totally surprised at the party and the number of people that cared and came, around 100 people.

A few Emails:

...I think you see the end of the tunnel now! Loved the pictures. What a handsome son you have Mr. Wilson...takes after his dad! I think you have the tiger by the tail there, hurry home
Susan S

...Jerry, just read your latest entry and I am so happy that Frank Dupont flew down to be with you. I know how close the two of you are, and there is nothing more comforting than to have an old friend by your side. In the meantime have fun eating your way through Amelia Island.
Helen R

...We have certainly enjoyed your journal as it gives such interesting insight into your experience. You are a man of many talents and writing is certainly one of your gifts. Just to make you feel good about your golf game, our 15 year old niece won the girls' junior North/South tournament this week in Pinehurst. 71, 73, 73 for a 5 stroke winning margin. We pray for you daily that the Lord will lay his healing hand upon you.
David & Diane A

...You talked about Andy Griffith in your journal, he taught me in Goldsboro High School...what a character he was. The other Bob.
Bob B

...Enjoyed your blog today. Louise taught and did a great job as always in Sunday school. Everyone is enjoying hearing from you. Hope BOB is not too bad in

the morning! We continue to pray for you, Jerry have a great week.
Becky J

…I loved the pictures. I saw Leona today in Sunday school and I told her you sounded good. You seem like you're having a great time. God can take something bad and make something good come out of it. You are living proof.
Allana G

…Listen 'Bo', you just having way too much fun, telling everyone you're under treatment. You just want to make us all jealous of golf and yacht clubs and great food. Take it easy, love ya.
Sue G

…Carol and I really enjoy reading your daily exploits. You are a gifted and entertaining writer, whose inspired genius falls somewhere between Henry David Thoreau and Dink Maness! Seriously, we love you and wish you God's continued healing.
Marshall F

…Just want to say that I am so glad your treatments are going well. It really sounds like God had his hand in getting you to the right place. Hope things continue to go well.
Susan E

…Hey beginner, you are wonderful…love how you write!!! So glad you had a fabulous day on the

links…wish I could have shared the day with you. I'm doing great, one day at a time, blessed each day.
Cynthia F

…I do love reading your journal. It's the highlight of my day. Does that tell you something about my life? I announced to the Sunday school class that you were lucky to have found ONLY my toothbrush. We will call again when you least expect it. Know you are in our daily thoughts and prayers.
Stafford C

…I read your latest commentary first thing every morning. That only goes to show you how hard up I am for entertainment! You are OUT OF CONTROL! I never realized before yesterday's column how much I owe my ministry skills to you. I feel like I'm hooked on a soap opera.
John C

…Congratulations Jerry. No doubt you are the worst speller in the United States. Sounds like you are doing well. Nice folks at Baxter's. Enjoying the blog.
Bill K

I appreciate your kind words and value your friendship. I don't normally advise wishing life away, but with you in Florida and my son in Afghanistan, I am praying that the day comes soon when I can see you both again. I love you, brother.
John C

…Just make sure you brush your teeth after eating the snails. Big time garlic! No kissing Frank Dupont.
John D

…You are computer illiterate. And when do you plan to join the PGA tour? And when do they plan to hang your photograph in Baxter's
Bill K

…Enjoyed as always…Escargots…well you are becoming quite the epicurean. It makes me hungry every time I read your journal.
Becky J

…Prayed for you and Frank Upchurch and the little baby today. Hope you are having a good day. I also have "Jesus Calling" it is a very good encouragement to you I am sure, as it always is to me.
Paula B

…Thanks for your kind words. We prayed for you and Susan Elkins at the end of our lesson. It is amazing to me that you are building others up while you are receiving these treatments. It is amazing that you can be so selfless. Jerry, you are more special than you will ever know. You have helped many of us to put our lives in perspective, both through Scottie's death, and your treatments.
Louise G

...Jerry, I really enjoy reading your day to day life. I know you will graduate from golf school and be home soon. Hope your day goes well.

George & Carolyn A

...I knew you would know everyone there in Florida before you came home!

Henry H

...Have a wonderful time with your friend. You are truly blessed to have such good friends. Play lots of golf and please figure out how to get us a new president!!! I will be interested in your findings.

Becky J

...You are priceless, thanks for sharing. I wish that I could come visit.
Susan B

...You sooo funny

Bill V

Letters:

A letter from **Danny Talbot**, maybe the best all-around athlete to ever come out of the state of North Carolina.

Jerry,

Just a note to say hello and let you know that you are in my thoughts and Prayers. Hope the treatment went well and look forward to hearing you are back to normal soon.

We have been friends for a long time and there is no doubt in my mind that being as competitive as you are, you will conquer this mess.

Danny Talbot

Frank Maynard, a childhood friend

Jerry,

Unfortunately, I am unable to be with you on this special night. Even though I'm not there in person; just know that I'm definitely with you in spirit. You made golfing and Baxter's sound so great, I am on my way to Amelia Island to enjoy…Just kidding. I have enjoyed reading your daily blogs, hearing about all the fun you were having with "BOB". Before I figured out who "Bob" was, I thought you were coming out of the closet…kidding. It sounds like you made the very best of a very challenging and difficult situation. I'm proud of you!

When I get back to Fayetteville, I look forward to catching up and perhaps maybe you can give me some of those golf lessons I read so much about in Florida. So glad you're back home with family and friends where you have been sorely missed.

From Rocky Mount, know that you are in our thoughts and prayers and we wish you the best of health going forward.

I happened to be with one of our mutual friends today and have attached a note from him (Danny Talbot), letting you know that he's thinking of you.

Take care and have fun,

Frank Maynard

Lauren Fuller, a friend who had allowed me to be grand dude to her daughter.

Jerry,

I think and pray for you daily and your courage to fight this disease, upbeat attitude, and overall love for life and for others is a quality that cancer can't take away from you. You have been an inspiration to our family as we battle the disease also. I have always loved you and Scottie, like y'all were my own. Also, Cool Kole loved meeting "Grandude", as she called you. I will forever cherish the fact that you met my daughter and took time to visit our family in Atlanta. I will continue to pray that health is on your side.
Sincerely,
Lauren Wallace

A sad note that Lauren lost her husband to cancer recently.

Doug Polk, childhood friend, we played a lot of baseball together growing up

Jerry,

Sorry I can't be there for your welcome home party. I am thinking of you and wish for your continued improvement in your health. By the way, BOB called and wanted directions....I sent him to Fayetteville, Arkansas!

Doug Polk

A little poem my son **Keith** wrote and read at the party...

Dear Jerry,

So long and farewell
My New and old friend
Please forgive me the discomfort
My presence did lend

Day in and day out
Is a fair description
Of our unusual relationship
They called a prescription?

My technique may be rough
My ways not so gentle
But my memory to you
Will always be sentimental

39 times we danced
Though I know you did not savor it

Of all the patients I've touched
Jerry, you were my favorite

Forgetting me soon
May not make you sob
But soon you will wonder
Who just met ole Bob?

This has been a tough year (For all of us) and I thank you for all your support of my Dad!

Thank you to Uncle Gary, and Aunt Beverly for helping put it together.

The owners here at Chris's (Greg & Luke) for helping us and being so accommodating with such short notice.

Thank you to my cousin Heather for putting a spark to this idea.

And a special thank you to Uncle Gary for buying my families dinner tonight!!!!

Allana Goodyear, good friend

Jerry,

Thank you for all the delightful stories, both truth and fairy tale. Your journals have enriched my life by showing me that cancer is not an automatic death sentence, that attitude is a big factor to healing, and that the spirit of the Lord is everything! Oh and that laughter is good medicine! May God bless and keep you and your family.

Allana Goodyear
Joe and Sandra Twiddy, friends from church

Jerry,
We are so disappointed that we will be unable to join you and you're "Welcome Home"! We will be in Raleigh for a week, dog-sitting our grand dogs while our children and grandchildren are vacationing in Florida! (Doesn't seem quite fair)

Thank you for sharing your "journey" with us. You will never know what an impact you have made on so many of us! You have shown true courage and determination, and hour humor has shown through it all. We are happy this journey is now behind you, and you can look forward to sunny days ahead!

Love
Joe and Sandra Twitty

Tim Finchem, Commissioner, PGA Tour (This is a joke folks, it's not Tim)

Dear Jerry

Congratulations!

It is my honor and distinct privilege to notify you of your PGA Tour playing rights for the 2013 season, based upon your remarkable completion of "Golf School" at Amelia Island.

Additionally, your acceptance of a PGA Tour player affords you full privileges to be a part of the Tour's annual "Pros in Swimsuits" edition, and our Board of Governors will be contacting you about your attire.

While you will be a rookie on tour, the board is seriously considering you for our centerfold, which would include a section dedicated to our new PGA line of Speedo's

Again, Congratulations,

Tim Finchem
Commissioner
PGA Tour

The following two letters were skillfully written by Bill Kirby, Jr. Bill writes for the local Fayetteville Observer newspaper and quite frankly, I'm amazed every time I read each of these letters. I will be forever grateful for Bill taking his time to do such a masterful job.

August 11, 2012

Dear John, (Jerry)

You left me without even a goodbye kiss.

I should have known.

We had, I Thought, such a personal relationship.

We were, after all, close.
I was deeply into you, you stinker.

I gave and never complained, letting you spend time with your friends Frank and Mike and Ray and Greg and your brother, Gary. Nor did I complain when you played golf all day, and then hung out all evening at Baxter's...night after night after night after night. I said nothing and just took it when you paraded along Fernandina Beach in your white Speedo.

I asked for so little.
Just 15 minutes a day.

And speaking of your brother, you may be twins...but he is so much better looking than you. I know that...*because he told me so.* If he told me once how much better looking, he told me twice and if he told me twice...and on and on and on. I do know this...he loves you dearly, more than his hair-dryer and his hair-spray.

And I thought you, my little Stinker, loved me, too

I know, I know, I know...you say that every time you turned around, it seemed like IU was up your behind. But only because I cared, you little Stinker.

I've been jilted before.

After all, you little Stinker, I've been places where no man has gone before. Alas, I have to accept it.

You, my love, have left the Island.

I wish you good health, and please understand that there is no wrath like a woman scorned...and I hope I never see your sorry behind, again!

With love and affection,
BOB

August 11, 2012

Jerry:
Welcome back!

All of us who have followed from afar your progress in these past eight weeks at the University of Florida Proton Therapy Institute in Jacksonville are inspired by your strength, and not to mention your wit and humor.

Most of all, your deep faith in God.
While I cannot be with you tonight, I hope that you will accept this journal – your journal – as you kept us apprised of your progress and treatment while in Jacksonville. Even with your own concerns, you always took time to think of others, from a grandson to a youngster you didn't know to an All-America, who means so much too so many in this city.

You made us laugh.

You made us cry.

You made us think.

"A journey with me" gives so many who confront cancer with hope for better and brighter tomorrow's and I know of the many hours and days you have spent at Cape Fear Valley Medical's Cancer Center encouraging others in health battles of their own.

"Jerry always brings laughter into the Cancer Center each time he volunteers or just visits, "Tara Hinton, coordinator for the Friends of the Cancer Center, was saying just the other day.

"He has been a volunteer for several years now, helping serve refreshment, assisting patients and families, and simply telling a joke to make them laugh. The only thing Jerry will not do...is wear socks."

She's got you there.

I know that your treatments will serve you well, and I know that your PSA numbers will indicate as much.

You are blessed with a loving family, and a brother who loves you dearly. And I need not say any more about your son and daughter, as I believe you will realize all the more tonight how much they love their father. And countless friends, again something you will realize all the more tonight. And finally, those two Guardian Angels...an angel named "Scottie" and an angel who goes by "Miss Rossie."

Again, Jerry, welcome home

Your Friend,
 Bill Kirby

Appendix A & B were written by Mr. Bill Kirby, Jr. and appeared in the local newspaper, The Fayetteville Observer.

Appendix A

Inasmuch as ye have done it unto one...

Scottie Wilson had a way about her. She put others before herself. She never forgot a birthday or a graduation or an anniversary.

Carefully, she selected her friends, and if she chose you, her friendship was unconditional and came without a price tag.

She had a strong work ethic, enjoyed a good book and had her own take on national politics. She didn't mind debating your view if you saw things from the other side.

She was a good judge of character, but she wasn't judgmental.

Her faith was strong. "She showed it through her actions rather than words" says Jerry Wilson, who was married to Irene Scottie Wilson for 44 years.

They met in the fall of 1966, students at Atlantic Christian College, now Barton University, in Wilson, and not far from her Rocky Mount hometown.

"We were married the following June 11, 1967," Jerry Wilson says. "People would say we had the perfect marriage, but no, I was the only imperfection."

Scottie Wilson would debate such a notion.

She loved her husband, a good man who has spent much of his time in the hospital rooms of Cape Fear Valley Medical Center, where his presence and encouraging words have meant much too many with health and cancer issues of their own.

Now, he struggles with the loss of a wife.

They shared so much together, a son and a daughter, three grandchildren, in-laws, nieces, nephews and so many smiles. Scottie loved to laugh.
"Scottie had three sisters that she was always crazy about," Jerry Wilson says. "Her sister Lee could make her laugh like no one else, I loved hearing them."

Scottie and Jerry Wilson were supposed to grow old together. They had plans.

There was the summer beach trip, just a couple of week's back, to be with the son she adored, and the grandchildren who lit up her brown eyes.

Irene Scottie Wilson died July 5, she was 65. "Her life," a grieving husband says, "was like a Bible verse..." Inasmuch as ye have done it unto one of the least of these."

Jerry Wilson gives pause.
"And this," he says, "She did!"

Appendix B

Cancer treatment strengthens his faith...

Once, he called on a woman who was struggling with a diagnosis of cancer.

"What are you doing here?" She snapped from her hospital bed.

He understood her sharp tongue, and her emotional state of mind.

"I'm here," Jerry Wilson told her, "because I have been right where you are."

He left the woman with a renewed hope that brighter days were ahead.

"Jerry Wilson has been a Friends of the Cancer Center volunteer for many years," says Brenda Hall, the center director.

A warm smile, she says, and a compassionate heart.

"Jerry has been a wonderful volunteer assisting patients, and families," says Tara Hinton, the center's volunteer coordinator.

"Jerry Wilson knows cancer, he is a survivor.

"I've been through the worst," he says, recalling the chemo treatments after being diagnosed in 1996 with Hodgkin's lymphoma, a cancer of the white blood cells.

"You wouldn't believe the hell I went through with Adriamycin.

He has been free of lymphoma for 17 years, but he was diagnosed in late March with cancer of the prostate…common in men older than 60. "I just want to live a normal life," says Wilson, explaining why he opted for a noninvasive treatment at the University of Florida Proton Therapy Institute in Jacksonville.

Well, sort of noninvasive.

Jerry Wilson might tell you there's a bit of encroachment when it comes to "Bob," the saline-filled balloon that stabilizes the bladder during the proton treatment.

"It sounds silly, but it's gonna be sad leaving this place," says Wilson, who underwent 39 treatments over eight weeks. "The people, the therapists, the technicians the nurses…all have been absolutely unbelievable." Jerry Wilson, 67, has shared his progress via my blog – The Gospel Truth – since June 17 in "A Journey with Me."

It's been a chronicle, replete with everything from his treatments to his appreciation for life to his unwavering faith to his infamous walk along Florida's Fernandina Beach in a white Speedo that frightened the sharks away and drove dolphins toward the Gulf of Mexico.

"We affectionately call Jerry "Job", because of the many challenges he has faced and overcome in his life," says the Rev. John Cook, senior pastor at Snyder Memorial Baptist Church. "He battled and beat cancer 17 years ago…He lost his precious wife, Scottie, unexpectedly last July. Any one of those events by itself could bring a man to his knees."

"Not Jerry."

"Not only has he weathered these storms with his faith intact, but he has been an inspiration to all of us, "Cook says. "He loves the Lord with all his heart, and Jerry knows it is God's grace that has brought him safe thus far."

Epilogue

Today, Jerry Wilson is back in this city he loves calling home, where he grew up along Rock Avenue under the watchful eye of Rossie Barnhill, a grandmother who taught him about a carpenter's footprints in the sand.

"What an awesome God!" Jerry Wilson has told us so often in his journal. "What an awesome God!"

On a very final note... The best thing we wish for in this life is to wish for GOOD HEALTH, and a BAD MEMORY.

Goodnight everyone, and may God Bless you all!

You see...there is a God!